Advancing Nursing Practice in Cancer and Palliative Care

Edited by
David Clarke, Jean Flanagan and
Kevin Kendrick

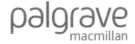

First published 2002 by
PALGRAVE MACMILLAN
Houndmills, Basingstoke, Hampshire RG21 6XS and
175 Fifth Avenue, New York, N.Y. 10010.
Companies and representatives throughout the world

PALGRAVE MACMILLAN is the global academic imprint of the Palgrave Macmillan division of St. Martin's Press, LLC and of Palgrave Macmillan Ltd. Macmillan® is a registered trademark in the United States, United Kingdom and other countries. Palgrave is a registered trademark in the European Union and other countries.

ISBN 0–333–77766–2 paperback

This book is printed on paper suitable for recycling and made from fully managed and sustained forest sources.

A catalogue record for this book is available from the British Library.

10   9   8   7   6   5   4   3   2   1
11   10   09   08   07   06   05   04   03   02

Printed and bound in Great Britain by
Creative Print & Design (Wales), Ebbw Vale

Dedication

As work on the book was being finished, our friend, colleague and co-editor Kevin Kendrick died suddenly and prematurely. Kevin was a devoted husband and father, a committed nurse and a dedicated writer and editor. He was also a passionate Liverpool FC supporter. Working on this book with Kevin represented many things. Editing this book was professionally satisfying, Kevin was instrumental in its initial development and contributed throughout the painstaking process of editing. As novices to the processes of book production it was rewarding to develop skills in this area in conjunction with a more seasoned editor. Like many other editors we would say that the process represented many months, indeed years of hard work and while this is true it somehow never felt like a chore. Most of all, the experience of editing this book with Kevin Kendrick was great fun. We are grateful for the time spent working together on this project.

David Clarke and Jean Flanagan

Contents

List of Figures and Tables

Preface

There is no doubt that the scope and nature of cancer and palliative care nursing is expanding and extending. The central aim of this book is to unravel the intricacies of extended and expanded practice in this field. As cancer and palliative care nursing is complex and related to the diverse needs and concerns of patients this analysis is broadly based. Thus, the contributions range from the technological aspects of care, to its moral, spiritual and ethical dimensions. Other contributions focus on family care and potential for expansion of the nurse's role in this important area. Chapters draw upon several different knowledge sources, both from within the domain of nursing science, where the application to cancer and palliative care is overt, to a broad range of other sources, philosophical, psychological and sociological. Advances in cancer and palliative care nursing are thus analysed from an informed and critical perspective.

The central theme of *Advancing Nursing Practice in Cancer and Palliative Care* relates to the highly contentious and deeply confused professional debate on the nature of 'advanced nursing practice' or 'higher level practice' within a specific context. Readers will quickly notice that the terms 'advanced', 'advancing', 'higher level', and 'expert' are used often and sometimes they are used interchangeably. Likewise the terms 'nurse-led' services and 'cancer nursing practitioner' and 'nurse consultant' are used as they describe particular advances in cancer nursing practices. We make no apologies for using this variety of terms throughout the book; we would welcome clarity of definition in these areas but do not see this as the purpose of this book. While we have sympathy with the view that the language used to describe nursing work is confusing, these terms are used in the everyday language of practising nurses and are also expressed as part of nursing policy. Moreover, these terms reflect the many ways in which professional boundaries are currently being re-negotiated in changing service provision.

While the book sets out a vision for advancing cancer and palliative care nursing practice, it also offers some direction on how to achieve that vision. Thus the final parts of the book are devoted to consideration of issues of leadership, management and policy. These elements are not only necessary but essential in order to make 'advanced' or 'advancing nursing practice' a reality.

We hope that you find this book useful, stimulating and challenging. We are deeply grateful to the many contributors who rose to the challenge in helping to articulate the ways in which 'advanced cancer and palliative care nursing' can contribute to patient care.

Notes on the Contributors

Gosia Brykczynska is International Nursing Consultant, International Department of the Royal College of Nursing.

David Clarke is Lecturer in Nursing, at the University of Leeds.

Gill Collinson is an independent consultant, and Programme Associate, at the Centre for Policy and Practice Development, University of Leeds.

Pauline Dodsworth is Senior Nursing Lecturer, University of Leeds and St Gemma's Hospice, Marie Curie Nurse.

Jean Flanagan is Education Development Manager, Macmillan Cancer Relief.

Anita Fatchett is Senior Lecturer (Nursing), at Leeds Metropolitan University, and a non-executive director, Wakefield West Primary Care Trust.

Janet Holt is a Lecturer at the University of Leeds.

Nic Hughes is Macmillan Lecturer, Macmillan Education Unit, at the University of Leeds.

Catherine Jack is Macmillan Lecturer, Macmillan Education Unit, at the University of Leeds.

Claire Kelly is Network Lead Nurse, with the Cancer Care Alliance, South Tees, South Durham and North Yorkshire.

Kevin Kendrick was formerly, Lecturer in Nursing, at the University of Leeds.

Chrissie Lane is a Network Lead Nurse.

Simon Robinson is Senior Anglican Chaplain and Lecturer in Theology, at the University of Leeds.

Susan Holmes is Director of Research and Development and Professor of Nursing, Faculty of Health, at Canterbury Christ Church University College.

Jean Steel is Professor and Chair, Advanced Practice Nursing, and Director, Centre for International Healthcare Education, Massachusetts General Hospital, Institute for Healthcare Professionals, Boston, Massachusetts.

Doug McInnes is senior lecturer in Research, Centre for Nursing Research and Practice Development, Faculty of Health, at Canterbury Christ Church College.

Part I

The modernising agenda for the National Health Services in the United Kingdom has a central notion that new working patterns will be created by motivated professionals who are appropriately experienced, educated and skilled. This is as true in cancer and palliative care services as it is in other services, and is a challenge faced by practitioners in other parts of the world. This part describes the current context of care, setting out in Chapter 1 the major changes and challenges for nurses as a professional group. The responses of the profession are then documented and analysed insofar as they demonstrate 'advancement in practice'. New practice innovations, for example the introduction of nurse-led services, are appraised.

Chapter 2 is a thoughtfully crafted account of the 'essence' of advanced practice as being fundamentally contained in the emotional and moral development of the cancer and palliative care nurse. It is argued that advancement in nursing cannot come solely from advanced technical skills and academic knowledge but must be accompanied by an 'advanced moral perspective and orientation'. Although challenging, this philosophical account of the qualities required of the cancer and palliative care nurse is highly pertinent.

Chapter 3 appraises the usefulness of 'nursing theory' for nursing practice. Advanced practice and advanced clinical decision making is formulated by using advanced knowledge, comprehension and understanding of core concepts. This theme is continued in Chapter 4 where the centrality of research to the advancement of practice is acknowledged and explored by Sue Holmes.

Part I

1

The Advancing Role of Nurses in Cancer Care

JEAN FLANAGAN, DAVID CLARKE, KEVIN KENDRICK
and CHRISSIE LANE

The past decade has seen many changes in the types of work undertaken by cancer nurses. Roles have become more diverse as new technologies such as biological therapies and high dose chemotherapy require nurses to extend their skills of assessment and supportive care. Some roles have become more technical with many cancer nurses taking responsibility for aspects of work such as the insertion of cannulae, the giving of chemotherapy, management of central venous lines and provision of specialist technical advice on symptom control. It could be argued that cancer nursing has become much more specialist, particularly following the publication of the Calman-Hine Report (Calman and Hine, 1995), with increases in disease specific posts such as lung nurse specialist and colo-rectal nurse specialists, adding to existing specialist posts such as breast care and palliative care. Nursing or rather individual nurses, have become more informed, as a growing number of both generalist and specialist cancer nurses have access to post-registration education and other forms of professional development. In many instances nurses are exercising more autonomy in patient management and this trend appears likely to continue. At the same time, nurses working in cancer and palliative care nursing must also respond to the calls in the NHS Plan (Department of Health (DoH), 2000a) for health professionals to overcome old fashioned demarcations between staff and develop effective teamworking in order to organise and deliver care based on the needs of the patient, rather than the needs of the service.

This chapter analyses the drivers for change which have impacted and will continue to impact upon cancer nurses as a professional group. Although it is probably never safe to make predictions, this discussion identifies the changing role of the cancer nurse, flexible working, nurse-led initiatives and the challenges presented by team working as the major issues with implications for nursing practice. Specific examples of innovative cancer nursing practice are used to illuminate and clarify the broader professional area of concern inherent in debates around advancing nursing practice. The nature and complexity of multidisciplinary team working is also examined in the chapter, it will be suggested that the concept of team working is uncritically accepted by health professionals. The modern health-care agenda demands new skills and new ways of working at an individual and team level and these issues will be considered as they impact upon the advancement of professional practice in cancer nursing.

The Changing Role of the Cancer Nurse

The beginning of the twenty-first century has been accompanied by healthcare reform. Inherent in the changing mandate for healthcare delivery is the assumption that new working patterns will be created by motivated professionals who are appropriately experienced, educated and skilled (DoH, 2000a, 2000b, 2000c, 2000d; UKCC, 1999). This modernising agenda is in turn driven by global, social and economic developments, sometimes characterised by social theorists as the changes associated with the development of a postmodern society. Conceptualisation of a postmodern society is widely considered to signal a qualitative shift in the nature of contemporary life. That is, that society has moved and indeed is moving, through a period of unprecedented change to become a different type of world altogether. The change can be likened to the change that occurred during the shift from a pre-industrial to industrialised society. Changes typically occur in every feature of life, its social structure, the economy, architecture, cultural media such as plays and television, and change in the nature and patterns of the types of work which people undertake. Nursing work is not immune from these changes.

A central feature of postmodern society is globalisation, the impact of which is significant and unavoidable. The South African statesman Nelson Mandela (2000) recently pointed out the futility of ignoring globalisation, likening it to stating 'I am not preparing for winter, when obviously winter is inevitable'. The main patterns of change in relation to work in a postmodern society and globalised economy described in the literature are:

- rise in information technology with competition for intellectual capital

- increasing core and periphery divisions in the workforce with a core of skilled technical elite and a periphery of lower skilled workers

- greater 'returns' from a flexible workforce

- patterns of 'upskilling' and 'multiskilling' leading to a breakdown in professional boundaries.
  (Bell, 1980; Lyotard, 1984; Crompton, Gallie and Purcell, 1996; Ride, 1997)

The job as characterised in the industrial revolution no longer holds true and work patterns will continue to change and blur as we move into this new century. Changes in professional boundaries can be observed in other professionals, with estate agents carrying out work more usually associated with solicitors, and some solicitors carrying out work previously done by barristers. Patterns of working in healthcare will continue to reform as successive governments in all industrialised nations face the challenges of providing high quality healthcare at a time of growing demand. The modernising agenda of current government policy sets out to face these challenges with major reconfiguration of the nursing workforce. Nurses are however no strangers to changing their role in relation to the changing needs of society. Contributing to this debate, a leading nurse educator has pointed out that if they had been resistant to change, then nurses today would not be recording blood pressure measurements, and health visitors would still be Salford Lady Sanitary Inspectors (Frost, 1998).

In recent years, many healthcare policy documents have been published, including *Making a Difference* (DoH, 1999), *The Nursing Contribution to Cancer Care* (DoH, 2000d), *A Health Service for All the Talents*, (DoH, 2000c), *Nursing, Midwifery and Health Visitor Consultants* (DoH, 1998), *A Higher Level of Practice* (UKCC, 1999) and *The NHS Plan* (DoH, 2000a). From these current policy documents two main themes emerge. First, that the agenda for change is potentially wide ranging and radical, and second, that there appears to be coherence across the many policies published. The emerging recurrent themes formative in the changing role of the cancer nurse are that:

- clinical work should be organised around the needs and preferences of patients. In cancer as in other services there is a need for timely and quality care
- there is a need to improve health, to save lives by preventing people becoming patients in the first instance
- there should be flexible working, to make best use of the ranges of skills and knowledge of staff
- along with flexible working there is a need for new, more flexible careers
- barriers, which say only nurses or doctors can provide particular types of care, should be 'done away with'

- there should be more emphasis upon working in teams across organisational and professional boundaries.

While the drive for changing the role of the nurse may appear to be centrally driven, it would be wrong, however, to imply that the nursing profession is, or has been, merely passive in determining its future direction. The nursing profession has worked diligently over many years to raise standards of patient care with the education and training of newly qualified and experienced practitioners. Cancer nursing as a specialist group of nurses, has been at the forefront of innovation and change within the nursing profession for over thirty years. In addition, in the United Kingdom, and in many other countries, the desire for acceptance of professional status has been a major dynamic in change. The tensions and perspectives within this struggle become apparent through labour force reform initiatives in the modernising agenda and the concept of flexible working.

Flexible Working and Flexible Careers: the Modern Cancer Nurse

The strategy for nursing laid out in *Making a Difference* (DoH, 1999), strengthens the nursing, midwifery and health visiting contribution to health and healthcare and sets out a proposed career framework providing a ladder of clinical opportunity stretching from the healthcare assistant to the consultant nurse. This model consists of different types of nurses and is congruent with Thornley's (1996) radical model of the ideal nursing workforce. The DoH's proposed strategy is more complex than previous outlines, and is characterised by a number of levels of nurses. This structure of healthcare assistant, registered practitioner, senior registered practitioner and consultant practitioner has greater flexibility than other models of the ideal nursing workforce. There is also more potential to deal with problems arising from professional barriers in healthcare.

The *Making a Difference* proposals are unlikely to appeal to the purist professionalisers whose model of the ideal nursing workforce is characterised by its search for professional closure associated with academic restrictions and attempts to define nursing as a profession clearly distinguished from doctors and ancillary workers. An example from the perspective of the professional model can be seen in an editorial of the *Journal of Advanced Nursing*, where two professors of nursing challenge the underpinning philosophies of the flexible career framework (Watson and Thompson, 2000). The radical model will undoubtedly be more appealing to the professionalisers than the traditional model which views less qualified, or unqualified, staff as equal to the registered professional nurse with continued acceptance of flexible boundaries across these differing groups of workers (Thornley, 1996). In the nursing workforce, Thornley identifies the 'nebulous character of skill' to be extremely problematic. This has resulted in grade dilution and consistent failure of nursing to 'achieve professional closure'; unlike, for example, 'midwifery', whose title is protected to those who are qualified midwives. Within the newly proposed career framework for nurses it is critical that the 'indeterminate nature of nursing skill' (Thornley, 2000) is articulated. Thus the competencies for cancer nursing must be made explicit and the system for monitoring and rewarding development of competence from healthcare practitioner to consultant practitioner must be made robust. These major challenges are being addressed on several fronts.

Changes to the career structure will necessarily impact upon the role of the nurse in cancer care, but such changes may be viewed as opportunities or threats. There is, for example, real potential for a life-long clinical career for cancer nurses with possibilities to combine or move laterally between practice, education and research. The opportunities here for careers, which are intellectually and financially satisfying are enormous and must be grasped by cancer nurses committed to take a lead in helping this occur. Unfortunately it is not uncommon for nurses in practice, education and research to view each other with suspicion or have a lack of mutual respect for the other's expertise. This should be addressed proactively by leaders in cancer nursing or there is a danger that such opportunities will be lost amid the quagmire of organisational politics and continuing clash of cultures. There is therefore a need for the cancer nursing profession to implement and evaluate models of working which support this clinical/academic career. The proposed new career framework undoubtedly heralds an increased supervisory role for the registered, senior registered and consultant practitioner. While there may be a determination to raise the status of practice based teaching as revealed in the *Making a Difference* (DoH, 1999) and *Fitness for Practice* (UKCC, 1999) documents, unless these initiatives are accompanied by resources, they are in danger of falling at the first hurdle (Manley and Garbett, 2000; Woods, 2000).

For some cancer nursing practitioners within a flexible career framework there is the prospect of holding greater responsibility and having more autonomy for clinical decision-making in clinical care. Thus the consultant nurse practitioner, for example, will be expected to:

- make and receive referrals
- exercise independent or delegated prescribing rights (where legislation permits)

- admit into and discharge from acute, community or hospice care
- develop nurse led clinics
- prescribe and initiate care/treatment packages in community and acute settings (DoH, 1999).

The consultant nurse and those operating at a higher level of practice are most likely to be those who are the driving and sustaining force behind role development and service development. Contemporary analysis of the advances in cancer nursing reveals the emergence of nurse led service initiatives. It would however, be folly to focus only on the changing and advancing role of nurses within the new NHS. Role redefinition and re-negotiation of role boundaries and function between professions is also a key concern for medicine and the professions allied to medicine. Between these disciplines the drive for effective teamworking is commendable but may be more complex than is suggested by the Department of Health (Miller *et al.*, 1999; ENB 2000).

Flexible Working: Nurse-Led Services in Cancer and Palliative Care

The draft document *A Higher Level of Practice* identifies that at a local level, healthcare professionals are determining the most appropriate way to deliver services. As a consequence of this, professional boundaries are becoming less distinct with nurses sharing and developing a skill base with other colleagues (Chapple *et al.*, 2000; Goodman, 1998; UKCC, 1999). These are currently best exemplified through several nurse-led services in cancer care involving substantial role developments. Role development has been described as the extension and expansion of the conventional nursing role (Lovett and Norwood, 1995). Within cancer nursing these services sometimes involve the extension and expansion of the psycho- logical support role of the nurse (Connolly and O'Neil, 1999; Moore, 1997); the supportive care function (Campbell *et al.*, 1997, 2000; Faithfull, 1999); rehabilitation (Guerrero, 1994, 2000) and the assimilation of work or services once carried out by medical practitioners (Guerrero, 1994; James *et al.*, 1994; Poole, 1996; Campbell *et al.*, 1997, 2000). The issue of role extension and expansion has been, and will continue to be, an area of contention within and without the profession, particularly as some see the denigration of the caring function to be related to such developments (Radcliffe, 2000). However, this trend toward role expansion and erosion of barriers between the professional groups is likely to continue. Lovett and Norwood commented that

Role boundaries are arbitrary and changing. At a time of workforce scrutiny, activity analysis and cost effectiveness, we should not be surprised that policy-makers and healthcare providers look to nursing to contribute to improving healthcare and health gain. It is not surprising therefore that role enhancement is seen as the natural opportunity (Lovett and Norwood, 1995).

These sentiments were echoed by the current government and were communicated directly by the British Prime Minister to the nursing profession in a special joint edition of the *Nursing Times* and *British Medical Journal* in 2000.

It means liberating nurses, removing unnecessary barriers ... There is no shortage of ideas on how bottlenecks can be overcome, delays reduced, services expanded and treatments made more effective. And we are determined that nurses will be the leaders of this change (Blair, 2000, p.15).

The discussion document *A Health Service for All the Talents* (DoH, 2000c) reveals one example of advances in cancer nursing practices.

We heard of a number of excellent developments in practice. In some places nurses are able to perform biopsies and clinical examinations when women are referred to the breast clinic. The nurse also continues to support the patient pre and post operatively being with, being with the woman through her treatment providing continuity and support (DoH, 2000c, p.3).

Other specific examples in the field of cancer nursing reveal that nurses provide a high standard of care to patients, which supports their expanded and developing roles. Moreover they appear to provide evidence that newly acquired skills are incorporated into the core of nursing's function and are not practised at the expense of psychological and supportive aspects of care. Three specific studies in cancer care demonstrate this. An evaluation of a nurse-led follow up system for neurological patients revealed that patient assessment by nurse specialists was satisfactory. Nurses encountered a range of problems that they were able to deal with as was demonstrated through analysis of consultation records. Audit demonstrated comprehensive patient assessments appropriate management and a decrease in medical outpatient workload by 30 per cent, in instances of nurse follow up of patients (James *et al.*, 1994). In a later study, a randomised trial was designed to evaluate the effectiveness of a nursing intervention in comparison to conventional medical care and demonstrated improvement in patient outcomes in a group with urological cancer (Faithfull, 1999). Patients expressed that they were more satisfied with nurse-led care than conventional care ($P = 0.002$) and valued continuity of care. The group had a reduction in some symptoms, for example, pain on micturition, although the differences in symptom experience were not great in the two groups. The study, which was a descriptive account of activities in doctor-led radiotherapy review versus nurse-led review, demonstrated a 31 per cent reduction in cost for the intervention group. Campbell *et al.* (2000) demonstrate that nurse-led care equates with quality care, and although nurse-led consultations lasted longest there was an overall reduction in waiting times in the service with its introduction. More interactions and activities were seen to occur during nurse consultations; for example, there were a greater number of referrals and liaisons with other support services leading to continuity of care. Of the 299 nurse-led episodes only 21 contacts were made with a doctor. Nurses dealt independently with the majority of concerns and problems raised by patients.

Advances across the broad remit of palliative care have also occurred offering commensurate opportunities for palliative care nurses to advance their practice, building and extending beyond the scope of those defining features mentioned so far within a multidisciplinary framework (Hearn and Higginson, 1998). This is particularly so in relation to pain management. Recent changes in the law relating to prescription of medicines will mean that nurses will increasingly have an advanced role to play in management of pain and symptom control when caring for people during the palliative process (Bagnall, 1996; Rycroft- Malone *et al.*, 2000).

However nursing defines advanced practice in relation to palliative care, there can be little doubt that practitioners will increasingly form part of the multidisciplinary team that prescribes medications for dying people. Beyond these elements, advancing practice in palliative care nursing also affords the opportunity to address pain and other symptoms through methods that can act as adjuncts to traditional pharmacological means. In this respect, complementary therapies offer a broad range of interventions that can help a dying person in relation to pain and symptom control (Penson, 1991; Kendrick, 1999). The following identifies just some of the complementary therapies that emerge from the literature:

- Abdominal massage in the treatment of constipation when there is no indication of intestinal obstruction (Emly, 1993).

- Therapeutic touch for physical, emotional and spiritual pains.

- Aromatherapy for agitation and anxiety (Gilliland, 1999).

- Reflexology to improve appetite, breathing, constipation, diarrhoea, fears of the future, pain, nausea, sleep, communication and tiredness (Hodgson, 2000).

It is hoped that such nurse-led developments in the realm of public health will be a force for change in reducing cancer-related deaths with, for example, cancer nurse consultants being a catalyst for the development and evaluation of successful interventions at the level of populations. There is a real opportunity here to demonstrate the worth of the cancer nurse in improving the nation's health and saving lives. A number of excellent examples spring to mind, for example in the implementation and evaluation of a teaching programme to help practitioners help people to give up smoking (Feber and Wilcocks, 2000). Another example shows how specialist practitioners can improve the access for populations to their scarce nursing skills. This is demonstrated by the partnership working of a school nurse and lung cancer nurse specialist in relation to the establishment of evidence-based health promotion interventions aimed at teenage schoolgirls, those most at risk of commencing smoking (Murray, 2000).

From the published studies available in cancer nursing it appears that nurse-led services are efficient and effective, and improve patient satisfaction. It is clear that these initiatives are not just concerned with delegation of roles but are concerned with changing the environment of care and putting patients' difficulties and problems higher on the agenda (Corner, 1999). Associated tensions with the term nurse-led services, particularly in a multidisciplinary context, are temporarily suppressed. This is because the term reflects one of the many ways in which professional boundaries are being re-negotiated in changing service provision. Nurse-led services mark a departure from terms used by nurses themselves, for example 'nurse specialist' or 'nurse practitioner', to demarcate boundaries and areas of work (Blackie, 1998). Extension and expansion of the nurse's role may indeed increase flexibility of employment and service delivery; however, there are associated risks from such patterns of employment and to be successful there needs be appropriate professional support. It is important also to recognise that role expansions are more likely to be accepted if there is multi-professional understanding of the potential benefits of role expansion and collaboration on the objectives of the service development proposed.

Flexible Working: the Need for Professional Support

One obvious tension in relation to notions of flexibility is simply that a flexible workforce may not necessarily be a happy workforce. The increased pressures on individuals to compete and be prepared to change their roles and established work patterns generates several issues involving stress. Upskilling and multiskilling nurses to achieve the flexibility required of them in the workplace may mean them experiencing a high degree of work related pressure. Evidence of an interesting relationship between skill change and work pressure is demonstrated by Crompton *et al.* (1996) through a comparative analysis of three large employment surveys. Questionnaire items were designed to indicate particular stresses and tensions associated with work; employees were asked for example how strongly they agreed with statements such as 'my work requires that I work very hard', or 'I work under a great deal of tension'. It was demonstrated that stress is least among those who have been de-skilled followed by those who experience no change in skill level. Employees who have some upskilling reported increased pressure, whereas those who have a significant increase in level of skill reported high levels of work pressure. Some nursing practitioners are responding to these increased demands at work but are part of a generation playing professional catch-up as educational goalposts are constantly being realigned. While many have shown great forbearance in balancing the drive for continuing professional development and taking more responsibility at work, it must surely be an urgent educational imperative to improve professional support for example using accreditation of prior and experiential learning (APEL) and work based learning (WBL) models of education. Use of APEL and WBL in education has enormous potential in harnessing the activities occurring within role and service developments, and making this count as currency in academic programmes (Flanagan *et al.*, 2000). As an approach to maximise opportunities for learning and professional development in the workplace and make them work toward an academic award, WBL has a clear advantage of avoiding duplication of effort. As an educational method it brings together the employee's knowledge and university learning, along with experience in the workplace.

Registered practitioners, senior registered practitioners and consultant practitioners of cancer care constantly engage in service and practice developments, and nurse education has now an opportunity to appropriately value such practice-based learning and support practitioners who are currently embracing notions of flexibility in their work. Professional competence is of utmost concern to the profession and to the public and such educational means have potential to ensure that the assessment of competence is robust. Professional competence is also in part supported and enhanced by the ways in which health professionals work together to deliver health services. The next section of the chapter will examine the nature of team working and will suggest that this concept needs greater critical attention.

Flexible Working: The Nature and Problems of Teamwork

So far in this chapter it is argued that cancer and palliative care nurses have an important role to play in developing and delivering services which will truly 'make a difference' to patients' lives. It is clear however that nurses are only one professional group contributing to the provision of modern health services. Most nurses will either work with or will collaborate with other health professionals in providing care as part of their daily work. There is a widely held view that multidisciplinary team working is likely to lead to improve patient outcomes and there is strong government support for this view at the present time (DoH, 2000c; National Audit Office, 2001). Essentially the argument is that in order to continue to deliver the healthcare agenda and fulfil the need for timely and quality cancer care, effective team working is essential. Although centrally important to best practice, working in teams across organisational and professional boundaries is fraught with difficulties, tensions, and inherent structural problems. The concepts of teams, team care and teamworking are so ingrained in the consciousness of most health professionals, that they rarely stop to question what is meant by the concepts, or whether teamworking is necessary or effective in the context of improving patient care. However as health services all over the world become more aware of the need to provide evidence to support the provision and delivery of services in specific ways, teamworking will come under increasing scrutiny and requires more critical examination. There is a widely held view that the outcome of care will be directly influenced not only by specific clinical interventions, but also by health professionals working together in teams. While it may be reasonable to assume that teamwork will contribute to improved patient outcomes, the relationship between the two has not been the subject of rigorous investigation. At present team working in healthcare cannot be claimed to be an evidence based activity (Strasser and Falconer, 1997; Schofield and Amodeo, 1999; Wilson, 2000). Major themes identified in the teamworking literature include, the failure to clarify and define terms in common use such as multidisciplinary, interdisciplinary, collaborative and transdisciplinary teams (Halstead, 1976; Ryan, 1996; Shute, 1997; Schofield and Amodeo, 1999). There is also considerable evidence that teamworking can be quite problematic (Evers, 1982; Luntz, 1985; Keith, 1991; Waters and Luker, 1996; Gibbon, 1999; ENB, 2000). It is important to note however that the limited number of critical reviews of teamworking in health and human services which have been published, do not appear to have made an impact on the popular consciousness of health professionals or policy-makers.

There is some uncertainty about what precisely is meant by team working in healthcare, and it may be that that because the concepts of teams and teamworking are so familiar to us, then detailed definition is simply seen as a semantic exercise of little value to the busy clinician. However, that clarity of definition can make an important contribution to understanding the nature of what health professionals claim as teamworking and more importantly, the potential relationship of teamworking to improved patient outcomes. In the context of this chapter the following definitions are adopted. A multidisciplinary team involves professionals from different disciplines who share a common task, for example working towards treatment or cure of an individual with cancer, or who are working with the same group of individuals, for example children with impaired physical ability. In multidisciplinary teams the common task is often based on or defined by the presenting disease or disability, for example head and neck cancer. The reason a multidisciplinary team is involved is that the presenting condition results in a complex clinical situation which requires expert knowledge and skills from more than one discipline. However, putting the individual disciplines together does not mean they will automatically function co-operatively (Miller *et al.*, 1999; ENB, 2000; Wilson, 2000). It is likely that many teams that work in this way pursue their own professional agendas first and foremost, and pursue team objectives second. Teamworking in this way may not have patient oriented goals as the drivers for care but may work towards uniprofessional goals.

Interdisciplinary teamwork implies that not only do team members perform activities towards a common goal but also that they accept the added responsibility of group effort on behalf of the patient (Garner 1994; Edwards *et al.*, 1997; Shute, 1997). According to Melvin (1980) 'this effort requires the skills necessary for effective group interaction and the knowledge of how to transfer integrated group activities into a result which is greater than the simple sum of the activities of each individual discipline. The group activity of an interdisciplinary programme is synergistic, producing more than each could accomplish individually and separately. In addition to the above it appears generally agreed that interdisciplinary teams are more likely to be effective because the individuals who make up the teams function as equals, with respect for the skills and knowledge brought by each. The team members will often contribute from differing perspectives (McClelland and Sands, 1993) but goal setting, care planning and decision-making are collaborative and shared activities, rather than led by a particular professional such as a physician (Garner, 1994; Shute 1997, Edwards *et al.*, 1997; Schofield and Amodeo, 1999). It is perhaps even more difficult to achieve effective interdisciplinary teamworking as this approach demands that team members overcome professional boundaries, status and hierarchical barriers and address the issue of power in the team, not a task for which most health professionals are prepared. This may be the way in which cancer and palliative care teams need to work with other health professionals to achieve the objectives outlined in *The NHS Plan* (DoH, 2000a).

The concept of transdisciplinary care appears to go one stage further than interdisciplinary care and involves team members functioning as equals, transcending team boundaries and engaging in carrying out the prescriptions of the other disciplines as part of the contribution to the therapy regime for a particular patient. An example of this would be where an occupational therapist, who was concerned with improving upper limb function post stroke, would use the opportunity presented by assisting a patient to eat a meal, to carry out the therapy for the upper limb function, but also to actively practice the prescriptions of the speech therapist in respect of assisting the patient with chewing and swallowing food. The significant movement on from the interdisciplinary model is the notion of shared skills. In the transdisciplinary approach, the team does more than share the decision-making, they share the implementation of the whole treatment plan and do not rely only upon specific disciplines to manage specific elements of the treatment plan. There are few examples of transdisciplinary approaches in the UK and US health professional literature; however, it is important to note that recent developments in the UK (DoH, 2000c) appear to be supportive of educating health professionals jointly in order that they can develop not only an understanding of each other's work, but also so that they can develop some core and generic skills which transcend existing professional boundaries. While there has been some blurring of health professional role boundaries in recent years, there seems little evidence at present that transdisciplinary teamwork is likely to become the dominant approach to team-based care in the short term.

Problems in Teamworking and Some Possible Solutions

There is little published research examining healthcare professionals' understanding of teams. However, a study conducted by Temkin-Greener (1983) challenged the view that the concepts of team and teamworking were well understood by doctors and nurses. More recent work by Cott (1997, 1999) in Canada also suggests that perceptions of the meaning and value of the multidisciplinary team held by team members differed, in part based on the professional background and status of the health professional, and on the level of contact with other team members. There may be more factors contributing to pulling teams in different directions than there are in pulling them together. Professional jealousies, professional role boundaries, power, status and gender, are issues which need to be considered in the context of preparing and supporting individuals to work in teams (Sands, 1993; Gibbon, 1999; ENB, 2000; Wilson, 2000).

All of these concerns must be considered and cannot be ignored by health professionals seeking to improve care for patients with cancer or long-term disabling illness. How effective teams are established is unclear; the evidence is they do not simply happen by imposing the team structure on professionals. At present almost all health professional groups in the UK receive their primary education largely separate from the other disciplines with whom they will later be expected to form effective work teams. The professional socialisation of these groups is within a unidisciplinary context. There are moves to address this problem (Miller *et al.*, 1999; DoH, 2000c; NAO, 2001), but without commitment and support from professional and educational leaders for initiatives such as shared interprofessional learning and shared foundation studies, there is no evidence that effective teamworking will be brought about. Both Miller *et al.* (1999) and the ENB (2000) suggest that particular approaches to learning and teaching need to be adopted if the potential of effective teamworking is to be realised. This involves much more than sharing the lecture hall for education in subject specific disciplines such as biology or pharmacology. It involves learning about teams, team functioning, managing conflict in teams and communicating effectively across professional boundaries. It is also likely that to begin to address some of the problems encountered in teamworking identified above, trainee health professionals will need to work collaboratively on clinical problems in ways that mirror the reality of professional practice (Miller *et al.*, 1999; ENB, 2000). For example, health professionals working in the fields of cancer and palliative care could work together to examine symptom management approaches for patients with chronic pain. Problem-oriented cases histories would be an appropriate medium for this collaborative educational activity, but this approach requires strategic planning by higher education and health service professionals responsible for health professional education. New healthcare commissioning arrangements with the shift from education consortia to education confederations from April 2001, provide real opportunities to realise this vision.

Conclusion

If the NHS modernising agenda is to be successful, then the challenges to health professionals in cancer and palliative care must be addressed. Nursing is continuing to respond to the need for the profession to develop its role and function in response to the changing needs and demands of the NHS. The examples discussed demonstrate nursing innovation, leadership and commitment to improving services. Issues such as flexible working, multidisciplinary teamworking and the drive for life-long learning are central to developing services which are expressly focused on the needs of patients. It is clear, however, that nursing, in continuing to expand and develop the profession, must also ensure that in maximising its contribution to multi-professional working, that the balance between uniprofessional concerns and those of other health professions is understood and addressed. In the future cancer care will present an enormous challenge for the health service. In order to provide the quality service which patients want and deserve there is a need for radical change. The evidence suggests that cancer and palliative care nurse are already responding to the challenge.

References

Ashworth, P. (2000) Nurse consultant – a role whose time has come. *Intensive and Critical Care Nursing*, 16, 61–62.

Bagnall, P. (1996) Don't overlook the real progress on nurse prescribing. *Nursing Standard*, 10(20), 10.

Bell, D. (1980) The Social Framework of the Information Society, in T. Foster (ed.), *The Microelectronics Revolution*. Oxford: Basil Blackwell.

Blackie, C. (1998) Community healthcare nursing in primary healthcare: a shared future, in C. Blackie (ed.), *Community Health Nursing*. Edinburgh: Churchill Livingstone.

Blair, T. (2000) Where you fit into our vision. *Nursing Times*, 15(96), 30.

Calman, K. and D. Hine (1995) *A Policy Framework For Commissioning Cancer Services*. A report by the expert advisory group on cancer to the Chief Medical Officers of England and Wales. London: DoH and The Welsh Office.

Campbell, J., L. German and D. Dodwell (1997) Nurse-led clinics in radiotherapy out-patient care. *Oncology Newsletter* (Yorkshire Regional Cancer Organisation), 20–23.

Campbell, J., L. German, C. Lane and D. Dodwell (2000) Radiotherapy outpatient review: a nurse led clinic. *Clinical Oncology*, 12, 104–7.

Chapple, A., A. Rogers, W. Macdonald and M. Sergison (2000) Patients' perceptions of changing professional boundaries and the future of 'nurse led' services. *Primary Healthcare Research and Development*, 1, 51–9.

Connolly, M. and J. O'Neil (1999) Teaching a research based approach to the management of breathlessness research in patients with lung cancer. *European Journal of Cancer Care*, 8(1), 30–36.

Corner, J. (1999) Cancer Nursing: a leading force for healthcare. *Journal of Advanced Nursing*, 29(2), 275–6.

Cott, C. (1997) 'We decide, you carry it out': A social network analysis of multidisciplinary long term care teams. *Social Science and Medicine*, 45(9), 1411–21.

Cott, C. (1999) Structure and meaning in multidisciplinary teamwork. *Sociology of Health and Illness*, 20(6), 848–73.

Crompton, R., D. Gallie and K. Purcell (1996) *Changing Forms of Employment, Organisations, Skills and Gender*. London: Routledge.

Department of Health (1997) *The New NHS: Modern, Dependable*. London: DoH.

Department of Health (1998) *Nursing, Midwifery and Health Visitor Consultants: guidance for appointments*. London: DoH.

Department of Health (1999) *Making a Difference: Strengthening the nursing, midwifery and Health Visiting contribution to health and healthcare*. London: DoH.

Department of Health (2000a) *The NHS Plan: A plan for investment, a plan for reform*. London: DoH.

Department of Health (2000b) *A Strategy for the Allied Health Professions*. London: DoH.

Department of Health (2000c) *A Health Service for all the Talents: Developing the NHS Workforce*. A consultation document on the review of workforce planning. London: DoH.

Department of Health (2000d) *The Nursing Contribution to Cancer Care*. London: DoH.

Edwards, J.B., P.E. Stanton and W.S. Bishop (1997) Interdisciplinarity: The story of a journey. *Nurse Healthcare Perspectives*, 18, 116–17.

Emly, M. (1993) Abdominal massage. *Nursing Times*, 89(3), 34–6.

ENB (2000) *Teamworking in Mental Health: Zones of comfort and challenge*. Research Highlights Report 40. London: ENB.

Evers, H. (1982) Professional Practice and Patient Care: Multidisciplinary teamwork in geriatric wards. *Ageing and Society*, 2(1), 57–75.

Faithfull, S. (1999) Randomised trial, a method of comparisons: a study of supportive care in radiotherapy nursing. *European Journal of Oncology Nursing*, 3(3), 176–84.

Feber, T. and T. Wilcocks (2000) *Implementation and evaluation of a teaching programme to help practitioners help people to give up smoking*, Clinical Directorate Conference, United Leeds Teaching Hospitals Trust.

Flanagan, J., S.A. Baldwin and D.J. Clarke (2000) Work based learning as a means of developing and assessing nursing competence. *Journal of Clinical Nursing*, 9, 360–68.

Frost, S. (1998) Perspectives on advanced practice: an educationalist's view, in G. Rolfe and P. Fulbrook (eds), *Advanced Nursing Practice*. Oxford: Butterworth-Heinemann.

Garner, H.G. (1994) Critical Issues in Teamwork. Chapter 1, in H.G. Garner and F.P. Orelove (eds), *Teamwork in Human Services: Models and applications across the life span*. Boston: Butterworth-Heinemann.

Gibbon, B. (1999) An investigation of interprofessional collaboration in stroke rehabilitation team conferences. *Journal of Clinical Nursing*, 8, 246–52.

Gilliland, I. (1999) Case report. Using aromatherapy as a therapeutic nursing intervention. *Journal of Hospice & Palliative Nursing*, 1(4), 157–8.

Goodman, I. (1998) Evaluation and evolution the contribution of the advanced practitioner to cancer care, in G. Rolfe and P. Fulbrook (eds), *Advanced Nursing Practice*. Oxford: Butterworth-Heinemann.

Guerrero, D. (1994) A nurse-led service. *Nursing Standard*, 9(6), 21–3.

Guerrero, D. (2000) Role of specialist nurses in follow-up cancer care. *Nursing Times*, 96(15), 15.

Halstead, L.S. (1976) Team Care in Chronic Illness: A critical review of the literature of the past 25 years. *Archives of Physical Medical Rehabilitation*, 57, 507–11.

Hearn, J. and I.J. Higginson (1998). Do specialist palliative care teams improve outcomes for cancer patients? A systematic literature review. *Palliative Medicine*, 12, 317–22.

Hodgson, H. (2000) Does reflexology impact on cancer patients' quality of life? *Nursing Standard*, 14(31), 33–38.

James, L., D. Guerrerro and L. Brada (1994) Who should follow up cancer patients? Nurse specialist based outpatient care and the introduction of a phone clinic system. *Clinical Oncology*, 6(5) 283–7.

Keith, R.A. (1991) The comprehensive treatment team in rehabilitation. *Archives of Physical Medical Rehabilitation*, 72, 269–74.

Kendrick, K.D. (1999) Challenging power, autonomy and politics in complementary therapies: a contentious view. *Journal of Complementary Therapies in Nursing and Midwifery*, 5.3, 77–81.

Lovett, P. and S. Norwood (1995) *Nurse Practitioners – Developments in England*. Paper presented to the English National Boards Annual Seminar, London.

Luntz, J. (1985) Some problems of being a professional on a team. *Australian Social Work*, 38, 13–21.

Lyotard, J.F. (1984) *The post-modern condition*. Manchester: Manchester University Press.

Mandela, N. (2000) Speech to Labour Party Conference, September 28th, Brighton, online archive web site: <www.guardian.co.uk>.

Manley, K. and R. Garbett (2000) Paying Peter and Paul; reconciling concepts of expertise with competency for a clinical career structure. *Journal of Clinical Nursing*, 9, 347–59.

McClelland, M., and R. Sands (1993) The missing voice in interdisciplinary communication. *Qualitative Research*, 3(1), 74–90.

Melvin, J.L. (1980) Interdisciplinary and multidisciplinary activities and the ACRM. *Archives of Physical Medical Rehabilitation*, 61, 379–80.

Miller, C., N. Ross and M. Freeman (1999) *Shared Learning and Clinical teamwork: new directions in education for multi-professional practice*. Researching Professional Education Series, 14. London: ENB.

Moore, J. (1997) Supportive models. *Nursing Standard*, 11(43), 26–7.

Murray, P. (2000) Preventing smoking in teenage children. Personal communication.

National Audit Office (2001) *Educating and training the future health professional workforce for England*. Report by the Comptroller and Auditor General: HC227. London: The Stationery Office.

Penson, J. (1991) Complementary Therapies, in J. Penson and R. Fisher (eds), *Palliative Care for People with Cancer*. London: Arnold.

Poole, K. (1996) The evolving role of the clinical nurse specialist within the comprehensive breast cancer centre. *Journal of Clinical Nursing*, 5, 341–9.

Radcliffe, M. (2000) How come we're losing if we scored the equaliser? *Nursing Times*, 96(15), 26.

Ride, T. (1997) The global challenge. *Nursing Times*, 93, 38–9.

Ryan, D.P. (1996) A history of teamwork in mental health and its implications for teamwork training and education in gerontology. *Educational Gerontology*, 22, 411–31.

Rycroft-Malone, J., S. Latter, P. Yerrell and D. Shaw (2000) Nursing and Medication Education. *Nursing Standard*.

Sands, R.G. (1993) Can you overlap here? *Discourse Processes*, 16, 545–64.

Schofield, R.F. and M. Amodeo (1999) Interdisciplinary teams in health care and human services settings: Are they effective? *Health & Social Work*, 24(3), 210–19.

Shute, R.H. (1997) Multidisciplinary teams and child health care: Practical and theoretical issues. *Australian Psychologist*, 32(2), 106–13.

Strasser, D.C. and J.A. Falconer (1997) Rehabilitation Team process. *Topics in Stroke Rehabilitation*, 4(2), 34–9.

Temkin-Greener, H. (1983) Interprofessional Perspectives on teamwork in healthcare: a case study. *Milbank Memorial Fund Quarterly*, 61(4), 641–58.

Thornley, C. (1996) Segmentation and inequality in the nursing workforce: re-evaluation of skills', in R. Crompton, D. Gallie and K. Purcell (eds), *Changing Forms of Employment: Organisation Skills and Gender*. London: Routledge, 161–81.

Thornley, C. (2000) A question of competence? Re-evaluating the roles of the nursing auxiliary and health care assistant in the NHS. *Journal of Clinical Nursing*, 9(3), 451–8.

United Kingdom Central Council for Nursing, Midwifery and Health Visiting (1999) *Fitness for Practice: The Report of the UKCC's Post Commission Development Group*. London: UKCC.

United Kingdom Central Council for Nursing, Midwifery and Health Visiting (1999) *A Higher Level of Practice*, Report of the Consultation on the UKCC Proposals For a Revised Regulatory Framework for Post-registration Clinical Practice.

Waters, K.R. and K.A. Luker (1996) Staff perspectives on the role of the nurse in rehabilitation wards for elderly people. *Journal of Clinical Nursing*, 5, 105–14.

Watson, R. and D. Thompson (2000) Recent Developments in Nurse Education, Horses for Courses or Courses for Horses? *Journal of Advanced Nursing*, 32, 1041–2.

Wilson, A.E. (2000) The changing nature of primary health care teams and interprofessional relationships, in P. Tovey (ed.), *Contemporary Primary Care: The challenges of change*. Buckingham: Open University Press.

Woods, L. (2000) *The Enigma of Advanced Nursing Practice*. Salisbury: Quay Books.

2

The Critical Essence of Advanced Practice

GOSIA BRYKCZYNSKA

Introduction

... Does the road wind-up all the way?
      Yes, to the very end.
Will the day's journey take the whole long day?
      From morn to night, my friend. (C. Rossetti)

Nursing patients who have been diagnosed with cancers and haematological disorders, and nursing patients who have reached the final stages of their disease processes, is not an easy or routine task. In fact, it is the rare privilege of a few select nurses to accompany these individuals on this difficult road. In view of the enormity of this task, not only is it imperative and a professional *sine qua non* that the cancer or palliative care advanced nurse practitioner be a specialist in their chosen field of practice, but it is crucial that he or she be an *exemplar* nurse. The advanced nurse practitioner is an exemplar professional who is not only a mentor to colleagues but also an expert support for patients and their families.

It is a privilege and honour to nurse cancer patients and those patients requiring palliative care, because in measure with the seriousness of the patient's received diagnosis is the obvious and concomitant rise in ontological and metaphysical questioning. As a result of such metaphysical questioning, there is an inevitable increase in humanistic reflection on issues of death and dying. Facilitating a patient's progress through this difficult yet essential phase in a person's life, is one of the greatest privileges that a nurse can ever expect to experience. Among the many tasks a nurse may be expected to fulfil, helping another human being to confront their humanity and human frailty, has no greater challenge and no greater reward. As many caring professionals have observed, it is the responsibility of the advanced specialist nurse to foster and encourage just such a nurturing atmosphere so that this essential human activity can take place within a humanising healthcare context (Stoter, 1997). As Simone de Beauvoir commented reflecting on her mother's death, 'There is no such thing as a natural death: nothing that happens to a man is ever natural, since his presence calls the world into question...'. The nurse's role in facilitating the patient to accept and understand this ultimate and inevitable of all human activities is awesome.

Patients and clients of the healthcare system are most in need of humanising and having their humanity reaffirmed precisely when their humanity and human existence is most likely to be threatened or apparently challenged. As the palliative care physician Sheila Cassidy rightly observed, 'One of the effects of the constant exposure to pain and death involved in the care of the dying is that one is forced to grapple not only with the "problem of evil", but with God himself' (Cassidy, 1988, p.65). To correctly interpret these intricate metaphysical moments in a person's life requires not only excellent technical nursing skills and academic prowess, that is, specialist competencies, but above all else it requires a certain *type* of nursing intervention, indeed, a certain type of nurse. The clinically effective and emotionally healthy advanced nursing practitioner in the field of cancer and palliative care practice, will be that nursing professional who has started to confront the nature of his or her *own* humanity. That is, the exemplar cancer or palliative care advanced nursing practitioner is that nursing specialist who has started to address some of the more pressing ontological questions and metaphysical arguments surrounding their *own* existence. That is, someone who has demonstrated the maturity and courage to feel comfortable in their work; an observation borne out by many counsellors, palliative care workers and members of the professional oncology community (Stoter, 1997; Campbell, 1984; Twycross, 1984; Cassidy, 1994). Indeed, the more comfortable a nurse is with his or her own humanity and human achievements, the more comfortable they will be with others and the more likely they will be to put others at ease, that is, to be truly therapeutic.

Advanced nursing practice in the context of cancer and palliative care requires a qualitatively different type of nursing intervention than simply a recognisable reflection and utilisation of an increase in cancer or palliative care knowledge and skills. This particularly doubtful approach is sometimes referred to as the *more-courses-the-better* approach. This approach implies the involvement of checking off the presence or absence of identifiable competencies and relevant nursing constructs, all of which have been gained or acquired through ever more complex nursing and academic courses, workshops and study days. The qualitatively different nature of advanced practice in cancer and palliative care, however, stems predominantly from a fundamentally different type of understanding of the *nature* of advanced cancer and palliative care nursing practice; rather than from a quantitatively larger pool of knowledge or even an increase in practical experience. Advanced practice involves such activities as fostering hope and promoting patient comfort when this is 'shattered', and having extraordinary courage in the course of a typical day's work, not just upon occasion (Morse *et al.*, 1994; Rees and Joslyn, 1998; Hauerwas, 1985, 1993).

This chapter addresses the ontological nature of advanced nursing practice in the context of cancer care, including palliative care, that is the critical essence of advanced practice. It illustrates the issues and areas that need to be confronted and addressed if the cancer and palliative nursing care that is being delivered is to begin to be considered as *advanced nursing practice*. The chapter concludes with recommendations and suggestions for the cancer and palliative care professional nursing community, which is attempting to introduce this complex notion of advanced nursing practice into their field of specialised work.

A Professional Ethic for Professional Care

> I am not lost and the way I followed has led me to the end – a barren land where pain
> is the fuel that slowly burns from the core of survival leaving an empty entity like the
> skulls of wildebeest turning into the essence of their creation ... (Stephens, 1990)

It is one of the paradoxes of human existence that in order to confront that which provides a common base for our mutual humanness, it is necessary to initially acknowledge the ontological reality concerning each individual's separate being. Thus, human individuals, through their very humanness unavoidably and necessarily demonstrate human uniqueness and the human essential and fundamental loneliness. It is this central human paradox that each person is similar to other persons to the extent that they are different, unique and unrepeatable that has concerned philosophers and theologians for centuries. Human individuals, who are otherwise correctly regarded as obligate social animals, are perceived ontologically as being unique individuals, or as Cicely Saunders poetically describes them – 'a community of unlike' (Saunders, 1990). In the Western philosophical tradition the human individual is considered most perfectly intact, when they have started to confront their own temporality, human fragility, and existential loneliness; that is, when they have started to acknowledge that they are not immortal, but necessarily imperfect. As the pastoral worker Henri Nouwen observed:

Many people suffer because of the false supposition on which they have based their lives. That supposition is that there should be no fear or loneliness, no confusion or doubt. But these sufferings can only be dealt with creatively when they are understood as wounds integral to our human condition ... (Nouwen, 1979, p.93)

In order to be recognisably sociable, the human individual needs first to confront his own uniqueness and metaphysical isolation from all other humans, just like all other humans have had to do, down the ages. Thus the human individual enters the world alone and exits the world alone. Needless to say, this is not the entire picture, for all along the human life trajectory, that is, from the point of a human's conception to the moment of death this essentially lonely human individual is *accompanied* by other human individuals. This is a paradoxical situation, that in order to be considered truly human one needs to go through a process of recognising and indeed defining oneself within the context of being surrounded by other human individuals. It is within this essentially human communal and social context of becoming human that the rare and beautiful privilege of professional nursing and midwifery occurs, a point beautifully brought out by the Australian nurse Beverley Taylor (1994). Because nursing practice is regarded as an intricate humanising art, which is practised by humans for the benefit of humans, it is even more significantly and essentially considered to be a *moral art*.

It is the honour of nurses and physicians to be designated by society the responsibilities of accompanying the human individual at the two most traumatic and potentially threatening moments of a person's existence, that is, the moments when a human first enters this world and when they prepare to leave it. Needless to say, nurses also attend to the various healthcare needs of humans at various other points in between these two pivotal ontological events. The sheer awesomeness of palliative care and the calculated ferocious audacity of cancer nursing, however, appears to put these two clinical nursing modalities in a category on their own. Nurses, however, represent only one of the many healthcare professions involved in cancer and palliative care work and teamwork is essential for the success of this work. As Philippe Poulain, editor of a palliative care professional journal recently noted, 'Staff working in this field have to recognise the fact that every other professional person, regardless of their position and rank in the management structure, provides an essential link in the palliative care chain ...' (Poulain, 1999, p.76). The moral art of nursing requires of nurses that they be aware of their interactions with colleagues in the multidisciplinary team and be cognisant of their all too human limitations but also the sheer breadth of their responsibilities, a point often made by cancer and palliative care nurses and physicians, such as Robert Twycross (1984), Sheila Cassidy (1994), and Lynn Brallier (1992).

The obvious question arises therefore, what are the unique *professional nursing* requirements for such a special and distinguished role as that of an advanced nursing practitioner, and what are the societal and *professional* requisites for such a clinician? Society entrusts these highly qualified cancer nursing professionals with protecting the seriously ill cancer patient from the worst effects of treatment, by buffering the patient from the effects of the disease and from the physiological and genetic misdirections and accidents that cancers and their treatments can produce. At other times society entrusts palliative care nurses with facilitating the ferrying of patients out of this world. What natural and acquired qualities are therefore sought after in the complex disposition of this highly privileged and multi-skilled individual?

As Ann Bradshaw (1994), a one time Macmillan nurse in the lecturer-practitioner tradition, demonstrated, since the very first years of professional nursing education leaders and teachers of the profession have been concerned with the moral, social and emotional development of nurses. From the very first attempts at professional nurse education in Europe and North America, it was recognised that professional nursing was not simply a matter of medical and nursing knowledge and accompanying specialist nursing skills but that it was also a matter of appropriate *disposition*. A good nurse was considered to be someone who actually approached and regarded the patient in a substantially different way not only from the physician but even from the patient's family. The professional nurse was someone who while not forgetting the inherent otherness of the patient was nonetheless capable of constructing therapeutic bridges between the vulnerable and ill patient and the 'healthy' care providers and family. These moral and social prerequisites in the professional nurse have been described in the professional literature of the past, but even more interestingly they have been described in the lay non-professional literature of yesterday and today. Given that nurses do not exist for their own ends or objectives but to service the needs of patients, that is, to service those in our society who are the ill, frail, wounded and disorientated, it is even more essential to consider what society itself seems to expect from the cancer or palliative care advanced nursing specialist.

Reading Leo Tolstoy's harrowing short story *The Death of Ivan Illych* (1960), one can well appreciate that what Ivan Illych required most during his long fight with cancer, was a thoughtful, efficient and competent palliative care nurse. But the profession of nursing was still in an embryonic state when Tolstoy wrote his famous tale, and the pioneering work of the hospice movement was not even a distant dream. It is all the more amazing therefore, that Ivan Illych's servant Gervasy was so sensitive and competent. Gervasy's insights and compassion should be carefully studied by palliative care nurses if they are to really come to terms with the soul of their work. If untrained lay individuals can deliver such flawless and excellent care, what are the implications for professionals, especially professionals who claim to be practising at an advanced level?

The therapeutic qualities required of the modern cancer healthcare worker have also been illustrated by the Russian dissident writer Alexander Solzhenitsyn. Again it is a lay person (albeit a former cancer patient, and therefore arguably the best type of cancer professional) who is stating what is required from the wise and compassionate healthcare professional. Solzhenitsyn (1969) in his epic autobiographical novel *Cancer Ward*, has Oleg Kostoglotov, the hero of the story, repeatedly dwell on the healing and restorative energies of Dr Vera Kornileyevna's gentleness. The physician's gentle disposition was perceived by Oleg as a powerful healing force, and in the estimation of Oleg wherever and whenever a similar gentleness was subsequently encountered, he thought of Vera, and was energised anew. By reflecting on the healing nature of Vera, Oleg's faith in humanity was restored, and he had something to live for once again. The power of this observation is noted most eloquently at the end of the narrative, when Oleg plans to meet up with Vera, once he is discharged from hospital, and realises too late that he cannot locate her. Upon reflection Oleg resigns himself to not meeting up with Vera (which is a complete turnaround from his hitherto firmly held plans). Oleg decided that he could live with this new and unexpected reality because despite not meeting up with her, he was still being empowered to go on living. Oleg realised that the good effect that Vera's all pervasive spirituality had on him was not limited to time and place but was of altogether another nature. The therapeutic nature of the professional encounter of Oleg the patient with Vera the physician managed to transcend the confines of physical presence and resulted in the permanent alteration of their casual physician–patient relationship and become something far more effective and long-lasting! This story is echoed in the parental grief expressed by Christopher Leach who observed about life and living that, 'It is a man's need to create. And other men, seeing creation, feel better able to live' (Leach, 1981, p.124) It was the creative art of gentleness as expressed by Vera, that made Oleg want to live and gave him the energy to continue living. It is therefore all the more interesting that when the moral philosopher Jean Porter, wished to present an analysis of a recognisable contemporary virtue she chose to analyse the virtue of 'gentleness'. As she noted, 'We all know, more or less, what it means to be gentle, and we can usually recognize a gentle person, a gentle voice, a gentle action or manner or way of doing something. Yet just what is it that we know, when we know what gentleness is?' (Porter, 1990, p.105)

Meanwhile, an example of the destructive nature of problematic dispositions encountered among health workers can be found in Simone de

Beauvoir's account of her mother's death from cancer in Paris (de Beauvoir, 1966). More so than in any other branch of healthcare, in cancer and palliative care nursing the person and moral disposition of the nurse is important and indeed crucial to a successful and beneficial patient care outcome. Unfortunately for the nursing profession, the nurses portrayed by Beauvoir were not too effective, in fact the writer went to great lengths with her sister to stop the hospital staff from *nursing* her mother...since they had such a detrimental effect on the elderly lady. The distraught woman pleaded with her daughters that they not leave her '..."in the power of the brutes" leaving Simone to reflect "...what agony it must be to feel oneself a defenceless thing, utterly at the mercy of indifferent doctors and overworked nurses...".

When contemporary Western society discusses the preferred disposition of nurses, the character traits which are most frequently articulated are those societal, cultural and moral constructs which include such characteristics as intellectual and technical competence, moderation, sometimes referred to as temperance, gentleness, courage, integrity, veracity, benevolence, humility, trustworthiness and so on. Needless to say, it is important to appreciate that these intra-personal qualities are to some extent culturally and socially determined, a point important to bear in mind, especially when discussing the transference of cancer nursing and medical practices to other parts of the non-industrialised and non-Judaeo-Christian world.

Meanwhile, Ann Bradshaw, in her splendid account of the spiritual roots of contemporary professional nursing in the Western tradition, makes the additional observation that the disposition of the nurse was always considered important to the founders of the nursing profession. It is not a new concern or a response to new problems. The early nurse educators did not separate moral, intellectual and practical approaches to patient care, and they assumed that the nurse would also reflect in her person a balance of moral integrity, spiritual awareness and intellectual acuity (Bradshaw, 1994, p.282). Since patients themselves were deemed to be in need of moral, medical and spiritual sustenance, that is holistic care, it is not surprising that nurses, too, were required to reflect a balance of these essential qualities in themselves. Moreover, these basic human and interpersonal moral dispositions considered to be essential for nurses, have already been described by generations of philosophers, theologians and pastoral workers as personal and interpersonal *virtues*. The ideal nurse in the estimation of the founders of modern nursing was always intended to be not only a competent individual but also virtuous person. Virtuous persons in turn have the ability to empower, enlighten and indeed to encourage others to become more human.

That contemporary society would like its nurses to reflect at least some of these personal and social, that is, other-regarding virtues should not be surprising. It is precisely because of the acknowledged inherent vulnerability and fragility of the patient that society demands of its nurses some measure of socially agreed upon moral, spiritual and social attributes. Henry Dom observes in a journal for palliative care healthcare workers, that

> Spirituality is concerned with transcendental, inspirational and existential way of living, as well as fundamentally and profoundly with the person as a human being, in relation to God and creation, Spirituality is normally heightened as the individual confronts spiritual pain and ultimate death of the human body (Dom, 1999, p.87).

Palliative care nurses care precisely for those individuals who may be in spiritual pain as they approach the 'ultimate death of the human body'. The palliative care nurse's work is intrinsically spiritual and existential in nature, as caring for individuals who are confronting their own humanness, existence and future non-being is an essentially ontological and spiritual pursuit, and needs to be facilitated by an expert in 'being human'; hopefully a good palliative care nurse.

Ann Bradshaw, citing the observations of Dr Cecily Saunders, the palliative care physician, notes that the underlying covenant relationship of healthcare worker and patient does not negate the existence of patients with 'maddening' ways. Indeed she says

> This covenant relationship does not assume an unrealistic or sentimental perfectionism in either the caring team or the patient himself... The ways of the individual, as Saunders writes, are often 'maddening'; patients, even when dying, can be difficult, just as nurses can be uncaring... Human being are capable of both great goodness and also great wretchedness... (Bradshaw, 1994, p.279)

It takes a morally developed individual to cope in trying situations, or find the reserves of therapeutic hope to share with others even when nursing the proverbial 'hopeless case' (Rees and Joslyn, 1998). Society does expect to see reflected in the nature of nursing and especially in the nature of the cancer and palliative care nurses' work a moral and spiritual dimension. Precisely because the essence of advanced cancer nursing practice is fundamentally an ontological and moral phenomenon, the effects of nursing therapeutic interventions rests on the cultivation of personal and professional virtues. Nurses are perceived by society as demonstrating an ethical approach to their work. They can be trusted to be ethical. It is for this reason that cautious elderly patients are prepared to open their doors to members of the healthcare team, even if they have never met them before, and anxious patients are prepared to confide in strange nurses, while fraught mothers will leave their children in the care of unknown paediatric nurses. In all these instances, society trusts the nurse to behave *professionally*, that is, society acknowledges the moral dimension of the nurses' labour and expects the nurse to respond accordingly. How irreversibly damaging it must be for the profession when nurses are subsequently found to be abusing the trust of elderly patients in the community, or that confidentiality is not being maintained or that children are being harmed while in the care of professionals (Pyne, 1998). As Maize-Grochowski (1984) noted almost twenty years ago, trust is fragile and once broken very difficult to build up again.

It is not so much the appropriateness or otherwise of society's desire to intervene and direct the nature of professional nursing which is primarily at issue here. The fascinating issue is the *nature of the rationale* for the desire by society (whom nurses serve and from whose pool of individuals nurses themselves are selected and educated) to see at least a minimum level of moral and emotional maturity among those who work as professional nurses. Society wishes to be assured that the ethical dimension of a nurses' work will not be neglected or lose its centrality in the complexities of modern practice. Contemporary society's preference for the existence of a virtuous professional nurse is the result of an attempt by society to safe-guard the interests of the vulnerable patient. It is not the intention of society to put extra constraints upon the efficacious and caring nurse, but society does want to be reassured that nurses will represent in their person a particular socially recognisable moral stance. What is most prob-lematic here, is that nurses themselves are not too sure what virtues if any they are to be collectively professing, that is, what is their moral nursing stance. Additionally, some nurses reflecting the growing trend towards moral relativism are so undecided about the nature of their own moral and social values that they understandably hesitate to articulate and therefore conceptualise necessary virtues for any professional nurse, not just for themselves.

At present nurses themselves define and determine the nature of nurs-ing practice and nursing professionalism. However, one of the greatest problems encountered with professions, is that after a while they start to lose touch with their socially determined roots and begin to serve their own interests, forgetting about those whom they were set up to serve in the first place. Reg Pyne (1998, p.8), writing for nurses in the United King-dom, notes that as far as he is concerned, 'the hallmarks of a profession is that it accepts the onerous burden of regulating itself, but recognises that this is to be performed for the protection of the public and not the prestige of its members'.

This is a point brought out quite clearly by Sharon Daloz Parks, in a paper she wrote in 1993. She adds to Reg Pyne's observations that, ' ... To have a profession is to have a stance, a way of perceiving and acting, held in common with and accountable to a community of others who bear like responsibility…'. This activity is even more difficult than in the past because

'… to have such a stance when we are all losing our balance. In this historical era, the young adult task of becoming an effective, responsible professional is dramatically more difficult because we live in a time of pervasive paradigmatic shift. The practice of trustworthy relationships – accountability – has become fraught with the tension between assumed patterns and emerging demands' (Daloz Parks, 1993, p.177).

Not only are schools of nursing entrusted with the academic education of nurses but they are also required by law to be satisfied as to the moral and psychological fitness of an individual to practice nursing. The assumed patterns of behaviours and emerging demands of society however, as to the idealistic profile of the professional nurse, is putting stress and strain on members of the profession. As Daloz Parks concludes, 'This tension is signalled in part, by the renewed activity around the issues of ethics and the professions over the past half dozen years' (p.177).

The recommendations of the Clothier Report should not be therefore considered that surprising. At the end of the special enquiry into the unfortunate happenings on the paediatric ward of Grantham General Hospital in the spring of 1994, the Clothier Report focused on the character of the prospective nurse. It looked at the need for character references required before an individual could be offered a position in the health service, the need for improved communication between schools of nursing and clinical placements and the need for more effective health screening procedures for new entrants into the profession, especially a clean bill of psychiatric health. In the wake of the Clothier Report, renewed emphasis was placed on the *person* of the nurse, not only the nurses' academic or professional qualifications.

It is vital that the profession of nursing work alongside society and not against society, if it is not to lose step with its patients and clients and the many frail and vulnerable individuals who require their care. We could say, that a nurse fulfils her specific role because society desires and requires the existence of just such a person who 'nurses'. Society in the United Kingdom wants and desires the presence of qualified cancer and palliative care nurses, as illustrated by the strong hospice movement and exemplary post-registration cancer nursing training programmes. An advanced nurse practitioner in cancer or palliative care nursing, is however no more of a *moral* nurse than the neophyte 'first-warder'. The advanced specialist nurse is equally accountable for his or her practice to the patient, society

and to the profession of nursing as a whole, in measure with their designated role in the healthcare team. In fact an advanced practitioner ought
to be an example of the wise therapeutic nurse, that is the nurse who is
competent and compassionate. For all these reasons, advanced nursing
practice is a highly skilled moral art, which has the curious property, that
the more it is practised, the more challenging, creative and *uncertain* it can
become. Nurses in palliative care and cancer work labour within a clearly
defined sphere of practical knowledge and practice, but in terms of their
moral obligations and ethical conduct, they remain fundamentally faithful
to the general nursing ethos which can be professionally demanding and
personally trying. Moreover, it is the universal nursing ethos, which
unequivocally supports the notion that as expert cancer and palliative care
nurses these specialists are ontologically bound by the very nature of their
work to demonstrate in their nursing practice a superior moral and spiritual stance.

If nurse leaders were concerned with the moral, spiritual and emotional
development of junior and student nurses in the past, not only about the
level of the students' academic knowledge and the adequacy of their
acquisition of specified nursing skills, the question might well be posed as
to what extent contemporary nurse educators and nursing leaders are
concerned with character-building virtues of practising nurses today? Some
nurses may even question how appropriate it is that at the dawn of the
twenty-first century leaders of the nursing profession and nursing educators should still be discussing the necessary professional *virtues* required
of the nurse, not to mention the virtues required for advanced nursing
practice. Such sentiments are certainly found in the current professional
press and some of their concerns are quite legitimate. In an interesting
paper, Winifred Pinch questions the sense of thoughtless rhetoric about
caring which can actually backfire and demoralise nursing staff: 'If nurses
are made to feel inadequate, unprofessional, immoral, or unsuccessful when
they are unable to care on a continuous basis, then caring is a devitalising
trap' (Pinch, 1996).

Other nurses argue, that these issues are concerns of the past and nurses
today neither behave uncouthly like Charles Dickens' Sarah Gamp or
unethically as nurse Rachett in the contemporary novel *One Flew Over the
Cuckoo's Nest*. For these nursing professionals, discussions about the moral
and spiritual qualities required of the advanced nurse practitioners are
considered to be a waste of time. Indeed for some nurses the unethical
component of their practice lies solely in the faulty nature of biotechnology,
medicine or market-driven pharmacology companies, but certainly not in
the nature of nursing practice *per se* which they consider to be inherently
good and therefore without fault or flaw. For these individuals, polemics
about the ethics of the profession of nursing are limited to discussions

concerning outside factors that impinge upon nursing practice, certainly not the intrinsic nature of the nurse him or herself.

Other nurses query whether the very debate about virtue and professional characteristics is itself not inherently flawed and potentially dangerous? They are afraid that discussion about the virtuous nature of the nurse can become an occasion for cultural or social bigotry and narrow-mindedness. After all, they say, perhaps swearing may be seen to be a cultural norm among particular members of our society and does not necessarily reflect the deliberate intention to harm anyone. They question why the profession (in the form of the UKCC) should designate swearing at patients as unethical conduct, *per se*? They are curious to know where does professional etiquette and moral aesthetics end and where does prejudice, bigotry and small-mindedness begin, and most importantly, does it and should it really matter and make a difference? Similar discussions have been noted in the nursing press concerning the wearing of jewellery, uniforms and various other socially determined professional phenomena. These are not trivial matters. It is well known that social and cultural norms do change over time, and that the interrelationship of professional and personal morality with culture and social norms is such that without constant vigilance moral attitudes and values can easily become skewed with changing social norms. Nonetheless it is also easy to see that under the guise of professionalism a lot of prejudice and bigotry can find a peaceful haven, which was one of the concerns of Winifred Pinch (1996). Such a situation would completely defeat the object of the cultivation of professional and personal virtues. Because some individuals misunderstand the object of virtuous living does not negate for others however, the lasting benefits from being truly virtuous.

Lastly, some nurses may doubt the need for such intense concern over the cultivation of virtues, in order to ensure the appropriate level of advanced nursing care. They query whether the profession of nursing needs to include the promotion and cultivation of virtues given the long list of requirements necessary for the demonstration of advanced nursing practice? They are not sure that the cultivation of virtues and the pursuit of practical wisdom are the critical essential ingredients in advanced nursing practice, without which there will be no effective nursing and certainly no sign of therapeutic advanced nursing practice? Nurses argue that while they want to see positive fruits of their labour and wish to work effectively and therapeutically, they do not feel that following down the path of virtue ethics will necessarily benefit them. They see this behavioural and moral approach as constituting a big undertaking, with uncertain professional and personal rewards. The question to be debated is does one really have to bother with personal moral development in order to be a better or a more therapeutic nurse?

It is not within the prerogative of individual nurses to start to disagree with the basic professional moral requirements set up with society and to try to impose upon society their own vision of the nature of the nursing profession. If our patients desire that we manifest a particular way of being, then as a profession we have no choice but to examine closely these societal propositions and only differ from them with good reason. Obviously nurses need to query where they are going professionally and why. Sometimes a profession may have a very good reason why it will present a different face to the public from that which is socially expected of them, but this needs to be done consciously and deliberately, not by default or because nothing better has been proposed. Indeed as Daloz Parks observes:

> Across all professions, the ethical norms of the past are now called under review. We are having to re-ask fundamental questions: What can be professed in a dramatically changing world? What is our ethical stance in the face of unprecedented problems and possibilities? Can virtue be taught? (meaning can the distilled wisdom of the present adult generation and its traditions be made usefully accessible?) and What virtues need to be taught? (meaning, What will constitute virtue in a dramatically changing environment?) (Daloz Parks, 1993, p.178).

Practical Wisdom the Perfect Nursing Virtue

The moral life depends on the quality of the images held at the heart's core. (Daloz Parks, 1993, p.182)

That caring is not a virtue in its self, can be argued, as Peter Allmark (1998) has demonstrated, but it can also be argued that fostering the presence of virtues, as understood by professional contemporary ethicists, should facilitate the flourishing of a caring mode of being, a point brought out by the nursing ethicist Marsha Fowler over fifteen years ago (Fowler, 1986). Moreover two of the 'professional virtues' that have been identified and shown to contribute to a professional state of caring and which have been taken on board by nurses and pastoral workers, are wisdom and compassion (Brykczynska, 1992, 1997). What is not yet clear, is to what extent the virtues of wisdom and compassion are sufficiently richly endowed of themselves, to be considered as self-sustaining virtues capable of promoting and generating holistic care; and to what extent they are only two strands (albeit very important ones) among many, in a much more intricately woven tapestry of virtuous care.

Virtue ethics and the interrelationship of wise living with a virtuous lifestyle is as topical a subject today for moral philosophers as it was several thousand years ago. Each age and period in human history corresponds to new attempts to redefine the essence of knowledge, virtue, and the nature of wisdom, and we are offered ever anew examples of the knowledgeable, virtuous, and wise person. But concepts of virtue, wisdom and the nature of science keep changing and as Jean Porter rightly observed:

> The connection between concepts of virtues and concepts of particular kinds of actions is obscured in many contemporary discussions by the relative lack of attention given there to the question of how we arrive at our notions of particular kinds of virtues (Porter, 1990, p.105).

When Porter proceeds to analyse the virtue of gentleness she starts to articulate the behavioural and affective prerequisites that we intuitively expect to find present in the 'gentle person'. She agrees with Stanley Hauerwas that a biographical narrative demonstrating a particular virtue should suffice to show what that particular virtue is about, since virtues are essentially by definition demonstrable 'moral ways of being' (Hauerwas, 1993). Thus she comments, 'we must be able to tell stories about persons whose lives exemplify that virtue' (Porter, 1990, p.108). It is not by accident that when Alexander Solzhenitsyn was defining the gentleness of Dr Vera he decided to do so by describing the physician's touch, her facial expression, the tone of her voice even the sound of her footsteps. He described in his novel the totality of the therapeutic experience resulting from the virtue of gentleness as *lived* by Vera Kornileyevna.

Using the example of one individual, Dr Vera, he managed to portray the essence of a particular virtue *in general*. If one cannot recollect a specific individual demonstrating a particular virtue, for example the virtue of professional courage, one needs to consider whether it is possible to imagine anybody manifesting that particular virtue, or is it humanly speaking, an unobtainable dream. If one can imagine a person demonstrating that particular virtue, that is, courage, even if one cannot name a specific living (or dead) courageous nurse, then that virtue of courage is considered to be humanly attainable and not simply the product of a rather florid imagination. Thus I can have in mind the nature of the essence of the virtue of courage which can be seen in the course of professional work, as was demonstrated by Edith Cavell and many a military nurse, even if I myself have never personally met a courageous nurse. This is important to the understanding of the nature of virtues, since while not everyone will be in possession of particular virtues this lack of seen virtues does not negate their intrinsic value, strategic influence upon human behaviour and thought patterns generally, and indeed very existence.

Aristotle, the ancient Greek philosopher, is considered to be one of the most influential philosophers from the past to write about virtue and the need to be virtuous. It is of practical interest to leaders of the nursing profession to ascertain to what extent contemporary nurses are indeed still guided by a virtue ethic as described by Aristotle and to what extent they are aware of the writings or thoughts of other more recent philosophers on this subject. Aristotle, the teacher of moral philosophy who lived in the fourth century before the birth of Christ, wrote extensively about the nature of virtue and being wise, most notably in his works *The Nichomachean Ethics* and *Eudomian Ethics*. Most contemporary discussion concerning the nature of virtue and practical wisdom pays some tribute to the role that Aristotle played in defining the virtues in these two works. His influence on subsequent moral philosophers and moral theologians was substantial, additionally so, since the medieval philosopher Thomas Aquinas re-interpreted and critiqued Aristotle's ideas for the Christian mind, and thereby considerably extending the lifespan of the Greek philosopher's influence on moral philosophy and popular morality.

For Aristotle, being wise, as demonstrated in practical wisdom consisted of many interwoven aspects of personal moral ways of being. Practical wisdom was considered by the philosopher to be reflected in a *combination* of moral characteristics and personal preferences (i.e. virtues) both innate and striven after. These characteristics included such ways of being as a functional practicality, the demonstration of at least ordinary intelligence, a capacity and potential for abstractness, an applied human shrewdness and above all else the presence of the fundamental underlying characteristic of moral reflection and insight. The last characteristic is often illustrated today by the presence of discernment and sagacity. Being wise, was perceived therefore by Aristotle to be the result of the combination of shrewdness and rationality, as would be evidenced in an instance of 'excellence in deliberation'; or in today's language, as would be reflected in effective thoughtful and fruitful reflection. It is interesting to note that the recommendation by nurse leaders for nurses to start practising *reflective practice* was one of the deliberately encouraged ways of enhancing and promoting advanced nursing practice.

Put another way, Aristotle considered someone to be at least potentially capable of being virtuous, first, if they were capable of demonstrating a common-sense approach to living and life in general (e.g. could sensibly prioritise tasks to be undertaken during the course of a shift etc.). Second, if they were capable of at least sometimes thinking in abstract terms, for example when nurses consider treatment options for patients; third, if they were not too gullible and naive and believed everything that they read and heard from politicians and managers; and fourth, were capable of reflection and moral discourse. All of Aristotle's conditions for being considered a virtuous person can be found in the preferred characteristics of a regis-tered nurse and are essential qualities of the advanced clinical expert nursing practitioner.

Aristotle considered practical wisdom to be crowned with a perception of morality that could be seen to be an *integral* virtue of just such a person who possessed 'wisdom' and therefore could be called both virtuous and wise. Thus, he claimed 'that it is impossible to be good in the full sense of the word without practical wisdom or to be a man of practical wisdom without moral excellence or virtue'. Indeed, Aristotle considered practical wisdom to be the *principle virtue* that binds together all other virtues, claiming that as soon as man 'possesses this single virtue of practical wisdom, he will also possess all the rest' (Aristotle, 1962, Book 6, Chapter 13, 1145a). A nurse for Aristotle (should the philosopher have had the pleas-ure of meeting one), would have been a good example of a person who at least in theory could be considered to be an exemplar candidate for the illustration of lived virtue and practical wisdom. The very job description of a good and effective nurse, that is the therapeutic nurse, is therefore considered to be congruent with the philosopher's definition of the virtuous and wise person.

For Aristotle, practical wisdom encompassed major universal concerns, and utilised the skills of deliberation in assessing these universal concerns. It was focused on human affairs and was entirely dependent on humane, morally good interpretations as might be achieved through contemplation of the morally good life and drew its strength of conviction from a reservoir of positive experiences. Finally, Aristotle pointed out the oft-stated truism noted by many psychologists even today, that '...a young man has no experience, for experience is the product of a long time. In fact, one might also raise the question why it is that a boy may become a mathematician but not a philosopher or a natural scientist. The answer may be that the objects of mathematics are the result of abstraction, whereas the fundamental principles of philosophy and natural science come from experience' (Aristotle, 1962, Book 6, Chapter 8).

It would be difficult to argue that a contemporary cancer or palliative care nurse should be anything else but an exemplar of Aristotle's practical wisdom. People with 'practical wisdom', according to Aristotle, have the '... capacity of seeing what is good for themselves and for mankind, and these are, we believe, the qualities of men capable of managing house-holds and states' (Aristotle, 1962, Book 6, Chapter 5).

If we consider the practical qualities required of the good practising advanced clinical nurse specialist, surely this 'practical wisdom' of which Aristotle speaks is one of the essential virtues we would cast aside at our professional peril. There is an element of caution, however, in Aristotle's consideration of practical wisdom, for he does not see it as a quality that can be entirely learnt or acquired or that we could train ourselves to acquire: 'It is not merely a rational characteristic or trained ability. An indication (that is something more may be seen) is the fact that a trained ability of that kind can be forgotten, whereas practical wisdom cannot' (Aristotle, 1962, Book 6, Chapter 5). Although wisdom and compassion are essential qualities for the advanced practitioner, there is a level at which these humanising qualities cannot be taught and cannot therefore be transmitted.

Aristotle saw the role of intelligence as necessary to 'apprehend' fundamental principles of science, scientific knowledge and *theoretical* wisdom, much as the profession of nursing requires evidence of a minimal level of intelligence from its practitioners to ensure the adequate interpretation of nursing data, facts and phenomena. Aristotle considered that intelligence should certainly be encouraged to flourish and develop, that is, he considered that there was a positive role for education to play, but that a personal quality was also necessary for the manifestation of true practical wisdom. This acquired 'intelligence' must be sufficiently internalised and absorbed by the nursing practitioner that it no longer can be regarded as transitory, whimsical, or a purely trained phenomena. The intelligence of the practically wise nurse is therefore a virtue, not only an academic intellectual asset.

For Aristotle, to be wise and virtuous was not just to display and possess certain moral characteristics, it meant *to actually be* a particular type of person, the *wise person*. If we saw nursing as a blending of philosophical insights and the re-interpretation of relevant theories from the natural sciences this eclectic interpretation might start to shed some light on the notion that practical wisdom in the context of nursing would take quite a while to develop. One does not start off by being the wise student nurse, but one may become, in time the wise expert practitioner. Thus, wisdom as perceived by Aristotle was a supreme virtue precisely because it represented an entire world-view and particular type or way of being that had been perfected over time and proven to be efficacious.

The English philosopher and essayist Francis Bacon (1516–1626) rightly puts scholarship into correct perspective as regards wisdom, when he commented that: 'crafty men condemn studies; simple men admire them; and wise men use them, for they teach not their own use but that there is a wisdom without them and above them, won by observation' (Bacon, 1952, p.150). The nurse practising at an advanced level would do well to remember this adage.

Philosophers such as Michael Slote (1992), physicians such as Sheila Cassidy (1988), pastoral workers such as Henri Nouwen (1980) and cancer nurses such as Louise de Raeve (1996), tend to agree that in order to be considered wise and virtuous individuals must have the ability to learn from what life presents to them and to have the ability to reflect upon life events. For this reason, while individuals can be taught the basic skills of nursing, for an individual to be considered as an expert practitioner and to be capable and competent to practice at an advanced level they would need to be additionally reflective. They would additionally need to be capable of correctly interpreting and *learning from* the many issues that daily living and professional work can throw at them. Otherwise these expert practitioners however advanced their preparation for their role, would never 'grow in wisdom', but they would ossify at the level of their last training and clinical experience, however sophisticated that might have been.

The need therefore for professional norms and ethical guidelines which would facilitate the discharge of ever more challenging duties (such as those of the advanced practitioner) are enormous, and much effort is constantly being put into updating and qualifying various codes of professional practice (Amnesty International, 1994). Meanwhile, no code of practice can ensure that a professional will actually appreciate the need to be conscientious, courageous, benevolent or just simply *wise*. Codes of practice work on a predominantly fear-inducing and a primitive deterrent principle, while virtue ethics attempts to *change* the very motivation and inclination of an individual towards perceiving and actually desiring that which is considered to be good. Promotion of professional ethics probably makes most sense, when a code of professional practice is augmented with an equally vigilant concern for developing professional virtues, as was noted by Daloz Parks (1993) in the context of business ethics.

Increasingly, contemporary scholars of philosophy are attempting to construct a model of virtue and virtue ethic, without the obvious and necessary recourse to ancient Greek scholarship. As noted previously, there are many problems in trying to discuss and define the nature of virtue for these academics, just as there were for Aristotle. As the contemporary moral philosopher Alasdair MacIntyre (1987) points out, times have changed, and what was considered a virtue in one country at one time, may not be necessarily regarded as a virtue by another people at another time. Even the significance and prioritisation of virtues can vary from individual to individual within a particular culture.

It is also rather dangerous to transplant wholesale ideas from one epoch and culture to another; for example, MacIntyre rightly points out the basic fact that is rarely acknowledged and therefore rarely elaborated upon by advocates of Aristotelian virtues, namely that for Aristotle the virtues which he wrote about were intended to augment the moral character of the educated man of State, never the slave or humble artisan (MacIntyre, 1987, p.119). Virtues were regarded by ancient Greek philosophers as moral dispositions attractive and peculiar to a particular ruling or warrior class. Above all, MacIntyre reminds us that when we are describing virtues and attributing authority for their definitions to ancient philosophers or even to more recent men and women of letters, it is crucial to understand the *context* in which these philosophers were living. It is crucial for a correct understanding of a virtue to understand what the definer of the virtue might have had in mind when advocating a particular way of life. Thus the practice of virtue can only be understood in the specific context in which the virtuous person is living. This truism was highlighted by William Prior and by many of the feminist writers commenting on contemporary applied philosophy. A virtuous nurse today will behave similarly to a virtuous nurse from the nineteenth century or even the twentieth century in some respects but in other aspects will differ quite substantially.

What is truly interesting is that MacIntyre at the end of his deliberations is convinced that it is possible to identify the presence of virtues in professional life and advocates the practice of these virtues even over many different cultures and in various contexts. In the context of nursing work, the question has been recently posed whether caring can ever be considered to be a 'true' virtue. The need to clarify whether 'virtue ethics' and 'caring ethics' share the same ideology and arguments is not difficult to understand. The very terms 'virtue ethics' and 'caring ethics' have been used recently by theoreticians and nurse ethicists almost interchangeably. Yet whereas virtue ethic has a long history of association with philosophical discourse, caring ethics is probably from its very inception a modern articulation of a particular virtuous way of being and the concomitant need stemming from this conviction to express this perspective through a particular professional stance. Needless to say there are shared ideologies between 'caring theories' and a 'virtue ethic', but there are also areas of differences.

When 'caring' theorists such as Neil and Watts (1991) take on a feminist paradigm or approach caring from a decidedly womanist stance such as in the case of Nell Noddings (1984), then the areas of overlap between the two philosophical perspectives of virtue ethics and caring ethics may indeed require a reconfiguration of the previously held common ground. Most crucial in this debate is an understanding of what is really meant by *virtue* and what is actually meant by the designation *caring*. It would be illustrative to know whether there are such identifiable 'professional' virtues for example, as nursing or professional caring or even whether there exist such character forming entities as womanly virtues, but these considerations will have to be discussed elsewhere.

Huston Smith (1993, p.18) reflecting upon these concerns makes the observation that while most modern thinkers locate the seat of knowledge in the head much like Aristotle, they also like Aristotle consider practical wisdom in some fashion to be a moderating influence on this head-based knowledge centre. Smith points out, however, that for many cultures and religions there is an alternative approach to the Aristotelian idea of the workings and focus of practical wisdom. He refers to a concept of 'heart knowledge', and considers that it is this 'heart knowledge' which moderates and educates the intellect rather than solely the presence of more reflection which is still an intellectual pursuit rather than a emotion, such as compassion. Smith is convinced that it is not so much the intellect that needs to be primed in order to be considered virtuous, as did Aristotle and many of his followers, so much as a need to 'open the eye of the heart'. This is perfectly in keeping with the current observations of many so-called caring philosophers and ethicists not to mention feminist philosophers who wish to see a more prominent place given over to the emotions in moral life and practical wisdom. This is a very contentious aspect of contemporary virtue ethics and the debate is still raging with the jury still out as to whether these contemporary philosophers are within the traditional virtue ethics fold or increasingly writing themselves out of it. What is clear, is that professional wisdom in the context of nursing must involve not only an intellectual component but also an emotional component, that is compassion. Without the presence of compassion it is impossible to talk about a caring professional or a wise professional nurse.

The crucial point to be made here is that nurses practising at an advanced level need to not only demonstrate advanced knowledge and technical skills but also an *advanced moral perspective* and orientation. Without this advanced moral orientation the advanced technical skills and academic knowledge will have no anchor or foothold or natural home in which to flourish. These newly acquired technical and academic attributes will be merely fancy additions upon a fundamentally unchanged that is, morally underdeveloped nurse. The moral orientation of the nurse in turn not only needs to reflect classical virtues – since this is what society expects from the nursing profession, but also an aspect of compassion, or as Alistair Campbell (1984) referred to it, 'moderated love'. The essence of advanced practice is the perfect balance of wisdom and compassion – of virtue and moderated love: that is, a caring mode of being; a professional reflection of personal morality and balanced emotions.

Conclusion

... *Where is the Life we have lost in living?*
Where is the wisdom we have lost in knowledge?
Where is the knowledge we have lost in information? (T.S. Eliot)

Many patients observe that their stay in hospital feels as if it were taken *out of time*, that it is *timeless*, or that they have *time on their hands* for the first time in their life, and just when they *know* what to do with *their time*, it is too late. There is not *enough time*. There is talk of time and timelessness, of too much time and stolen time. Indeed, life has become for them a form of timeless waiting, waiting to resume life, or waiting for the end of life, or most crucially, waiting to make sense of life. As the Bishop said to Mark, the young curate in Margaret Craven's semi-biographical account of life among the Indians of the Pacific North West, we need to live only as long as it takes to learn 'enough of the meaning of life to be ready to die' (Craven, 1967, p.119).

Moreover, C.S. Lewis in *A Grief Observed*, comments that not only life but also grief can be considered to be akin to a type of waiting. He notes that grief consists of

> ...hanging about waiting for something to happen. It gives life a permanently provisional feeling. It doesn't seem worth doing anything. I can't settle down. I yawn, I fidget, I smoke too much. Up till this I always had too little time. Now there is nothing but time. Almost pure time empty successiveness (Lewis, 1961, p.29).

With all this time and waiting and anticipating and postponing patients have the resources to observe and evaluate the medical and nursing staff in quite cruel and minute detail. Fortunately most patients are satisfied with the care that they receive and most nurses are satisfied with the care that they deliver. But in order to maintain this fortunate situation the leaders of cancer and palliative care nursing need to constantly scrutinise their practice and to work at ongoing self development and increased moral sensitivity. The critical essence of *advanced* practice in this field of nursing is the ability to acknowledge the awesomeness of the human individual and to stand in professional and personal humility before the wonder and splendour which is the human spirit. The essence of this practice is not only to acknowledge one's humanity but to embrace it and help others to become more human. As one patient commented, 'I, the unwilling recipient of the title of being human. The very logic of the word sends despair and a desire not to participate in the beginning to the end sequence' (Stephens, 1990, p.9) Advanced practitioners of cancer nursing need to get behind these bitter and angry words and reaffirm the human way of being 'in the beginning to the end sequence'.

If this interpersonal quality and virtue of humility in face of wounded humanity is lacking, however, then no amount of courses and degrees in cancer nursing will make an advanced practitioner out of a cancer nurse technician. It is ironic that to be considered an advanced professional prac-titioner in this field of work requires from the nurse the acknowledgement of a common universal human frailty, an openness to the wonder and a fundamental joy but also pain of being human – a truly wise attitude.

These human responses result from the internalised truth that the caring human mode of being is one of mutual reciprocity and concern, and in turn is energising and fulfilling for the wise practitioner (Roach, 1984). The critical essence of advanced cancer and palliative care nursing is a *wise nursing attitude* which is in turn sustained by concerted professional compassion and competence. As Tolstoy noted in his epic saga *War and Peace*, 'The highest wisdom has but one science – the science of the whole – the science explaining the whole creation and man's place in it' (Part V, Chapter II) Advanced nursing practice is such a *science of the whole*. A holistic practice demanding of the specialist practitioner an understanding of the whole human course of being. It demands of practitioners' knowledge about being human. The essence therefore of this professional holism in advanced cancer and palliative care nursing practice is a deliberately nurtured and cultivated virtue of practical wisdom. Advanced cancer and palliative care nursing needs wise practitioners to move the profession forward – nurses who are competent and compassionate, nurses who care about being human.

References

Allmark, P. (1998) Is caring a virtue? *Journal of Advanced Nursing*, 28(3), 466–72.

Amnesty International (1994) *Ethical Codes and Declarations Relevant to The Health Professions: An Amnesty International compilation of selected ethical texts*. London: Amnesty International.

Aristotle (1962) *Nichomachean Ethics*. Indianapolis: Bobbs-Merrill.

Bacon, F. (1952) *Essays*. London: Dent.

Bradshaw, A. (1994) *Lighting the Lamp: The spiritual Dimension of Nursing Care*. London: Scutari Press.

Brallier, L.W. (1992) The Suffering of Terminal Illness: Cancer, in P.L. Starck and J.P. McGovern (eds), *The Hidden Dimension of Illness: Human Suffering*. New York: National League for Nurses, 203–25.

Brykczynska, G. (1992) Caring – A dying Art? in M. Jolley and G. Brykczynska (eds), *Nursing Care: The Challenge to Change*. London: Edward Arnold, 1–45.

Brykczynska, G. (ed.) (1997) *Caring: The compassion and wisdom of nursing*. London: Edward Arnold.

Campbell, A.V. (1984) *Moderated Love: A theology of professional care*. London: SPCK.

Cassidy, S. (1994) *Light from the Dark Valley: Reflections on suffering and the care of the dying*. London: Darton, Longman & Todd.

Cassidy, S. (1988) *Sharing the Darkness: The spirituality of Caring*. London: Darton, Longman & Todd.

Craven, M. (1967) *I heard the owl call my name*. London: Picador.

Daloz Parks, S. (1993) Professional Ethics, Moral Courage and the Limits of Personal Virtue, in B. Darling-Smith (ed.), *Can Virtue be Taught?* Notre Dame IN: University of Notre Dame Press, 174–5.

de Beauvoir, Simone (1966) *A Very Easy Death*. Harmondsworth: Penguin.

de Raeve, Louise (1996) Ethical Commentary, in L. de Raeve (ed.), *Nursing Research: An Ethical and Legal Appraisal*. London: Bailliere Tindall, pp. 103–17.

Dom, H. (1999) Spiritual care, need and pain – recognition and response. *European Journal of Palliative Care*, 6(3), 87–90.

Fowler, M. (1986) Ethics without virtue. *Heart and Lung*, 15, 528–30.

Hauerwas, S. (1985) Virtue, in K. Vaux (ed.), *Powers that make us human: The foundation of medical ethics*. Urbana: University of Illinois Press, pp. 117–40.

Hauerwas, S. (1993) The difference of virtue and the difference it makes: courage exemplified. *Modern Theology*, 9(3), 249–64.

Leach, C. (1981) *Letter to a Younger Son*. London: Arrow.

Lewis, C.S. (1961) *A Grief Observed*. London: Faber.

MacIntyre, A. (1987) *After Virtue: a study in moral theory*, 2nd edn. London: Duckworth.

Maize-Grochowski, M. (1984) An analysis of the concept of trust. *Journal of Advanced Nursing*, 9(6), 563–72.

Morse, J.M., J.L. Bottorff and S. Hutchinson (1994) The phenomenology of comfort. *Journal of Advanced Nursing*, 20, 189–195.

Neil, R.M. and R. Watts (eds) (1991) *Caring and Nursing: Explorations in Feminist Perspectives*. New York: National League for Nursing.

Noddings, N. (1984) *Caring: A Feminist Approach to Ethics and Moral Education*. Berkeley, CA: University of California Press.

Nouwen, H.J.M. (1979) *The Wounded Healer*. New York: Doubleday.

Pinch, W.J. (1996) Is Caring a Moral Trap? *Nursing Outlook*, 44(2), 84–7.

Porter, J. (1987) Perennial and Timely Virtues: Practical Wisdom, Courage and Temperance. *Concilium*, 191, June, 60–8.

Porter, J. (1990) *The Recovery of Virtue: the relevance of Aquinas for Christian ethics*. Louisville, KY: Westminister/John Knox.

Poulain, P. (1999) The professionalism of palliative care personnel. *European Journal of Palliative Care*, 6(3), 76.

Pyne, R. (1998) *Professional Discipline in Nursing, Midwifery & Health Visiting*. Oxford: Blackwell Science.

Rees, C. and S. Joslyn (1998) The importance of hope. *Nursing Standard*, 12(41), 34–5.

Roach, S. (1984) *Caring: The Human Mode of Being*. Perspectives in Caring – Monograph 1. Toronto: Faculty in Nursing, University of Toronto.

Saunders, C. (ed.) (1990) *Beyond the Horizon: A search for meaning in suffering*. London: Darton, Longman & Todd.

Slote, M. (1992) *From Morality to Virtue*. New York: Oxford University Press.

Solzenitsyn, A. (1969) *Cancer Ward*. New York: Strauss & Giroux.

Smith, H. (1993) Educating the intellect: An opening the Eye of the Heart, in B. Darling-Smith (ed.), *Can Virtue be taught?* Notre Dame, IN: University of Notre Dame, pp. 17–32.

Stephens, J. (1990) *Read my Mind: Statements, stories and poems from the heart of a haemophiliac with AIDS*. Dublin: Kildanore Press.

Stoter, D.J. (1997) *Staff Support in Health care*. Oxford: Blackwell Science.

Taylor, B. (1994) *Being Human: Ordinariness in Nursing*. Melbourne: Churchill Livingstone.

Tolstoy, L. (1960) *The Death of Ivan Illych*. New York: New American Library.

Tolstoy, L. (1957) *War and Peace*. Volumes 1 and 2. London: Penguin.

Twycross, R. (1975) *The Dying Patient*. London: Christian Medical Fellowship.

Twycross, R. (1984) *A Time To Die*. London: Christian Medical Fellowship.

3

Beyond the Theory–Practice Gap: the Contribution of Theory in Nursing

DAVID CLARKE

Introduction: A Restricted View of Theory in Nursing

Mentioning the words 'theory' or 'nursing theory' to many nurses results in any of a number of reactions ranging from raised eyebrows and facial grimacing, dismissive and or derogatory comments, through to sceptical or cautious interest. For many nurses their experience of theory in nursing has been the exposure to the writing of North American nurse theorists such as Peplau (1952, 1988), Roy (1984) and Orem (1970, 1995). This exposure has usually come during the completion of educational programmes at pre-and post-registration level, and until recently, has focused almost exclusively on being introduced to nursing models and attempting to apply these models to their own area of clinical practice. The application has either been required formally as part of an assignment, or has taken place informally as an exercise in examining ways to improve the nature and organisation of practice in a particular clinical setting. Initial interest in the conceptualisations of nursing expressed by nurse theorists has often been followed by frustration for many clinical nurses as they have been exhorted to 'use a model of nursing' in practice but found the model could not adequately support or develop their practice.

Until recently nursing models themselves were seen as above criticism, implying that the problem of a mismatch between local nursing practice and a nursing model must be due to the practice or the practitioner. However, not all nurses have had negative experiences of theory in nursing, and there are some good examples of where nursing theory has been positively embraced and appears to have contributed to the development of practice in a given setting. The groundbreaking developments at Tameside in the 1980s (Wright, 1986) and at Burford during the 1980s and the 1990s provide good examples of this (Pearson, 1992; Johns, 1994). McKenna (1997) suggests that nurses sometimes adopt an anti-intellectual stance when it comes to learning about theory in nursing and the new language which accompanies theory. This anti-intellectual stance related to theory in nursing is often in stark contrast to the willingness of nurses to learn complex new words and terms associated with pathophysiological processes, treatment modalities and pharmacological interventions. Some of the reasons for this apparent contradiction will be now be explored.

This chapter argues that for too long nurses and nurse educators have held or been taught a restricted and narrow view of theory in nursing. This narrow and restricted view has largely ignored the rapid change and development which has occurred in nursing and healthcare over the past ten years. It has also failed to convey the developments in nursing knowledge and nursing theory in ways which would capture the attention and interest of nurses. Theory in nursing must do more than be a vehicle for enhancing the academic and professional standing of nursing, it must have practical utility and be actively and critically examined by nurses seeking to enhance and develop patient care. Theory in nursing must also have utility in contemporary health services that are characterised by technological advancement, economic stringency, blurring of boundaries between primary and secondary care and a growing concern with the experiences and rights of patients as consumers of healthcare. In order to argue that a broader and more positive view of theory in nursing is required to truly advance practice in cancer and palliative care nursing, this chapter examines the nature of knowledge and theory in nursing and briefly reviews the recent literature on the theory practice gap in nursing. Factors affecting nurses' perceptions of the utility of theory for practice will be explored. Advanced practitioners in cancer and palliative care nursing must be able to make clinical decisions on the basis of advanced knowledge and comprehensive understanding of the care and treatment options available to the patients and families they work with. This advanced level of knowledge will include theoretical knowledge as well as proven factual information. Both these forms of knowledge contribute to the collection of responses available to nurses in cancer and palliative care. The final section of the chapter argues that nursing practice and theory in nursing are inextricably linked, and that the development of one is contingent on the development of the other.

The Nature of Knowledge and the Nature of Knowledge for Nursing

The debate surrounding the nature of knowledge and what can be known (epistemology) has occupied philosophers for over two thousand years. The discussion here focuses on contemporary discussions in relation to nursing, but the reader is asked to consider that these debates are common to most academic disciplines and have more than an academic relevance to the discipline.

Part of the narrow and restricted view which has dogged theory in nursing is that until recently there has been a relative absence of examination and debate about the nature of knowledge and theory in nursing. Two important questions which have been examined in detail in the academic nursing literature, but not necessarily in nursing education and practice, are first, *what is* nursing knowledge, and second, what knowledge do nurses *need* to practice effectively (Donaldson and Crowley, 1978; Carper, 1978; Emden, 1991; Chinn and Kramer, 1995). At the most basic level we can regard knowledge as 'the awareness or familiarity gained by experience of a person fact or thing' and also 'the theoretical or practical' understanding of a subject, for example language' (*Concise Oxford Dictionary*, 1990). Knowledge required for professional care giving clearly has some association with knowledge gained in everyday human experience. It is generally accepted however, that professionals are expected to have additional or extended knowledge on which to base their practice. Thus knowledge can be seen to be gained from experiencing a situation, for example being in pain. This has been referred to as *the process of knowing*. Knowledge can also be gained by being taught factual information, for example that naturally occurring endorphins can mediate the pain experience of individuals. This has been referred to as *the product of knowing* (Chinn and Kramer, 1995). These authors differentiate between knowing and knowledge, knowing is referred to as the individual human process of experiencing and comprehending the self and others in ways that can be brought to some level of conscious awareness (process). Knowledge however, is defined as what can be shared or communicated with others (product). Chinn and Kramer (1995) and others (Manley, 1997; McKenna, 1997) note that a hierarchical view of knowledge has emerged in which objective, formal or scientific knowledge became the most highly valued, both by members of Western societies and also by nurses as health professionals within those societies. This view explains in part why knowledge of pathophysiology, pharmacology, immunology and biochemistry has gained a highly valued position in education programmes for nurses in cancer and palliative care. Critics of the scientific view have pointed to the value of other forms of knowing which have been termed subjective, personal, intuitive, informal or tacit knowing (Freire, 1972; Rogers, 1983; Schön, 1983; Benner, 1984; Rolfe, 1996). These forms of knowing have gained popular support in the nursing literature in the past 20 years.

Visitainer (1986) suggested that the knowledge base for a discipline could only be defined following separation of that knowledge which was important for the discipline and that which was not. In this chapter and throughout this book the various authors have engaged in selecting out knowledge that they consider is important for nurses involved in advancing practice in cancer and palliative care. It is argued in this chapter, that the process of separating out the important knowledge for the discipline has only become deliberate and logical in the past 25–30 years. Prior to that time much of what was believed to be important for nursing was defined, either by those who were not part of the discipline for example medical doctors, or by default, in that what nurses did defined what nurses needed to know. Examples of the latter can be seen in the curriculum content of post-registration diploma (e.g. ENB 237) and degree programmes focused on cancer and palliative care nursing. The selection of content for many of these programmes is driven in large part by what nurses providing cancer and palliative care are doing in practice settings at present, or are predicted to be doing in the near future. An examination of the content of these programmes indicates a major emphasis on the disease process, on pharmacological, radiological or combined chemotherapeutic interventions. More recently the psychological sequelae of cancer or chronic illness have rightly gained a higher profile. While this selection of content may be there mainly because it reflects the daily practice of nurses, it is generally considered appropriate by nurses working in these specialist areas as the knowledge can be seen to have utility in increasing their understanding of patients treatment and can thus contribute to the provision of nursing care. In general nurses do not reject the inclusion of the knowledge and theory on which these subjects are based because it is considered to add to the nurse's own knowledge and understanding and to have practical utility.

However, content related to nursing knowledge and theory has often been included because the syllabus from National Boards required it, or because nurse educators felt that nursing programmes could not be claimed to be such unless they contained nursing theory. Thus in many instances nursing theory, in the form of the nursing process or nursing models was delivered to nurses as facts to be learned and then applied to practice. The historical traditions of submission to those in positions of power and authority in nursing led most nurses to respect the authority of the professional regulatory bodies and of nursing's academic and professional leaders. It was (and perhaps still is) accepted that they would determine what knowledge was important for the discipline (Rolfe, 1996; Rafferty, 1998). In the late 1970s and the early 1980s, few nurse educators were prepared to critically evaluate and argue for alternative forms of knowledge for the discipline. Recent policy documents (DoH, 1999) have attempted to shift the focus of selection of curriculum content away from an educator dominated activity to a partnership activity, where the needs of healthcare providers and consumers are more closely reflected in the content of programmes. However, uncritical acceptance of nursing theories is one factor that led to frustration for both practising nurses and nurse educators. Some of this uncritical acceptance can be seen to be a result of the educational preparation of nurses. Until 1989 this was based largely on development of practical or technical skills, the teaching and learning of an agreed set of responses or procedures required to provide care for patients with certain medical diagnoses, and the general require-ment for an acceptance that those in positions of authority held know-ledge that it was not really appropriate to question.

Despite the well intentioned aims of Project 2000 to educate nurses to be knowledgeable doers (UKCC, 1986) and many well developed pro-grammes of post registration education, there is little evidence that nurse education programmes have truly prepared nurses to think critically and to develop the skills of evaluation and analysis (Clarke and Holt, 2001). These skills do not result from simply completing programmes in higher education institutions but must be actively developed by educators and students (Glen, 1995; Chenoweth, 1998). Nurses have come to expect nursing theory to be part of their programmes of education, but these programmes do not appear to have prepared nurses to be able to critically evaluate the nature of knowledge needed to practice nursing in different settings or to view nursing theory as being anything other than nursing models. It is not surprising therefore that they have rarely been able to see the utility of nursing theory for their practice.

What Sort of Nursing Knowledge is Useful for Practice?

Chinn and Kramer (1995) suggest that in a human science such as nursing it is necessary for both formal, scientific, informal and subjective know-ledge to contribute to the body of knowledge in the discipline. It can be argued that in the fields of cancer and palliative care, nurses encounter individuals who often have the double burden of complex and life-threatening disease, together with the unique psychological and spiritual challenge of adjusting to a diagnosis of cancer or chronic disabling disease. Knowledge for nursing practice in these situations cannot be based on formal scientific knowledge alone. The most well-known discussion of ways of knowing that need to be utilised in nursing is Carper's 'patterns of knowing' (1978, 1992). Carper (1978) examined nursing literature and identified four patterns of knowing. The following section will attempt to examine each of the forms of knowledge identified by Carper in order to illustrate how each may make an important and integrated (but not often consciously examined) contribution to the skilled daily practice of advanced practitioners in nursing.

Carper's (1978) Patterns of Knowing

- Empirics: the science of nursing
- Aesthetics: the art of nursing
- Personal knowing: knowledge of the self
- Ethical knowledge: moral knowledge in nursing

Empirical knowledge is commonly equated with scientific knowledge, which is highly valued both by the public at large and by healthcare professionals in general. Traditional scientific approaches have been closely associated with underlying (empiricist) assumptions about truth and reality, which are that there exists an objective reality, independent of the observer, which is waiting to be discovered. Thus the function of scientists is to systematically investigate the natural world in order to discover knowledge that can be organised into general laws and theories. These laws and theories typically develop through the development and testing of hypotheses or statements about the world, whose truth can be confirmed by experimentation on, and observation of, the world. This approach has formed the basis of knowledge generation in sciences such as biology, chemistry, physics and mathematics. In medicine the randomised controlled trial has become the gold standard for making statements (or true claims) about the most effective forms of treatment for certain diseases. The ultimate goal of empirical investigation is to produce knowledge that allows the scientist to describe, explain, predict and control the world. Thus the decision of the physician to prescribe treatment A as opposed to treatment B can be claimed to be on the basis of scientific evidence (objective reality) of its efficacy as opposed to a personal belief, a historical tradition, or the view of an individual in authority.

While this form of knowledge is acknowledged as being an important and necessary component of knowing in nursing there is also the concern, or criticism, that scientific approaches in the empirical tradition fail to account for the full range of human experience. Thus it is accepted that the effects of a particular drug on specific cell surface receptors or specific genetic or biochemical processes involved in cellular reproduction can be objectively measured. However, there is also the acknowledgement that while this (empirical) knowledge may be valuable in predicting the post-treatment prognosis of a particular disease, it often cannot account for the differing human responses to treatments which have been shown to be effective in scientific trials. Chinn and Kramer (1995) suggest that this is because understanding human responses to disease, health and illness requires knowledge which is based on more than an objective view of individuals as collections of cells, tissues and organs, but is also based on knowledge which accepts that individuals experience complex and dynamic interactions between their physical, psychological, social and spiritual worlds.

Carper (1978) suggested that the nurse theorists writing in the 1950s, '60s and '70s were strongly influenced by the empirical tradition. This can clearly be seen in the description of assumptions, concepts, propositions and theoretical relationships in the writing of Henderson (1966), Neuman (1982) and Roy (1984). However, the nursing models or theories developed by these authors did not develop through the approach of hypothesis testing, but by what Cody (1996) has termed a 'black bag approach' (p.88). Cody's criticisms were based on a concern that this approach reflected an unspoken acceptance that nursing was an applied discipline only, and thus it was appropriate to borrow knowledge from other disciplines without seeking to utilise this knowledge in ways which would grow and sustain the body of knowledge which nursing could claim as its own. For Cody then, empirical knowledge is relevant but must be synthesised in the context of nursing actions rather than simply applied. In addition to a focus on empirical or scientific knowledge, nursing models attempted to account for the influence of the environment, personal beliefs and values and individual experiences. In including these other factors, which the authors maintain have an effect on the person's experience of health and illness, nurse theorists clearly acknowledge the need for forms of knowledge other than empirical to be reflected in the knowledge held by nurses.

While empirical knowledge typically deals with factual information where a correct answer or response can be selected, nurses and other health professionals frequently find themselves dealing with situations where questions arise for which there is no single satisfactory or correct answer. In these situations ethical knowledge can make a major contribution to the ability of the nurse to respond to the complex moral dilemmas which arise in the context of provision of individual, family or community care. Carper suggests that ethical knowing encompasses 'an understanding of different philosophical positions about what is good, what ought to be desired; what is right' (1978, p.20). Nurses and other health professionals often have to make difficult and rapid judgements about what actions to take to safeguard or protect the interests of individuals or their families or, on occasion, colleagues with whom they work. These decisions can be more confidently made when there is a knowledge and understanding of formal ethical principles and ethical theories. Ethical theories cannot provide specific instructions regarding how to act in a certain situation, which can be claimed to be the case with empirically derived theories. The value of ethical knowledge is that it can provide the basis on which nurses can examine the merits of the alternative actions available to her. This will often include a commitment to respect the rights, values and beliefs of those in her care, and to clarify the reasons for selecting one course of action from a range of sometimes imperfect alternatives.

Ethical knowledge can be examined separately from other forms of knowledge in the course of learning about ethical theories but in reality nurses will often draw upon other forms of knowledge when engaged in clinical decision-making. For example, consider the complex situation of working with a patient who plans to refuse a specific treatment for his form of cancer. The recommended treatment, although unpleasant at times, may have been shown in randomised clinical trials to improve prospects of five-year survival by up to 30 per cent. Adherence to ethical principles requires that the nurse examine alternatives which ideally, will do most good for the patient, or at least will do no harm. In addition the right of the individual to express his personal beliefs and to exercise choice about what he wishes to happen to him should be respected. It is not difficult to accept these principles, but the nurse and other professionals must balance this ethical knowledge with the empirical knowledge gained from clinical trials. In supporting and caring for the patient, the nurse in this case would be faced with the knowledge that the patient's decision may not be in his best interests in terms of treating his cancer. However, we have made the case earlier in this chapter that the patient is more than a body within whom there has developed cellular abnormality resulting in cancer. Providing support and care in this case requires examination of not only empirical and ethical knowledge but also what Carper (1978) termed *personal knowing* and *aesthetic knowing*.

In the past 15 years there has been a growing acceptance that personal or self knowledge is an important part of what the nurse is able to bring to her interaction with a patient. The work of Macleod-Clark (1984), Neeson *et al.* (1984), Burnard (1985), and Bond (1986) in the United Kingdom was influential in raising the profile of communication skills, self awareness and self understanding in nursing. While there are teaching and learning strategies which can help nurses develop an understanding or awareness of self, this form of knowledge is not factual and cannot be taught *per se*. Rather, personal knowing involves the ways in which nurses see and feel about themselves. It is the process of developing an understanding of the dynamic and changing awareness of self. Personal knowing encompasses a knowledge of one's beliefs and values and the factors which have shaped and continue to shape these, it also involves the recognition that we grow and develop as a result of our experiences within and outside of nursing. These experiences contribute to our knowledge and under-standing of self which is influential in our actions and interactions with others. Chinn and Kramer maintain that 'it is through knowing the self that one is able to know another human being as a person' (1995, p.9). The notion of therapeutic nursing and the therapeutic use of self (Carper, 1978; McMahon and Pearson, 1995) is founded upon personal knowing, where the nurse consciously uses her knowledge and understanding of self and an openness to expressing and sharing her experience of self in interaction with patients. In our example of the patient refusing treatment the nurse's personal knowing will contribute to her ability to know the patient as another human being, and to develop meaningful understanding of his beliefs, thoughts and anxieties in the context of his specific situation at this point in his life. The nurse's ability to acknowledge and examine her own beliefs regarding coping with cancer, taking decisions about one's own life, and her understanding of the meaning of the patients actions will be in part dependent on her personal knowing. Thus personal knowing will be integrated with empirical and ethical knowledge and will guide the nurses actions with and for the patient.

Closely related to personal knowing is the form of knowing which Carper termed aesthetics, which is also referred to as the art of nursing. If we think of a continuum of knowledge from at one end the scientific, objective, factual and measurable to at the other end the subjective, intui-tive and situation specific, then aesthetic knowledge can be found at the latter end of the continuum. The art of nursing is not easily expressed in words or language but finds expression in the actions, bearing, conduct, attitudes and interactions of the nurse in unique and specific situations. Chinn and Kramer (1995) suggest that aesthetic knowing is what makes it possible for the nurse to know immediately what to do at a particular instant or moment, without conscious deliberation about the alternatives. This form of knowing can also 'transform the immediate encounter into a direct perception of what is significant in it' (Chinn and Kramer, 1995, p.11). Carper (1978) believed that the perception of meaning in an encounter is what creates an artful nursing action, with the nurse's perception of meaning being reflected in the action she takes in the specific encounter. To regard the art of nursing as simply 'gut' reactions is to ignore the complex reality of nursing actions in specific interactions with patients. The concept of aesthetics has been expanded by Chinn and Kramer, who identify that aesthetic knowing involves three linked creative processes. These are engaging, intuiting and envisioning. Engaging requires the direct involvement of the self within a situation which allows one to fully experience the moment. Intuiting is regarded as the process by which meaning is perceived in the situation. This perception of meaning derives from the nurse's unique subjective experience and knowledge which is interpreted in the context of the patients unique human experience. Intuiting leads to creative responses to the patient's situation, to what is called envisioning the actions or responses needed to bring about the most appropriate intervention or interaction required at this particular moment. Benner (1984) and Benner and Tanner (1987) have undertaken research related to the nature of expertise in nursing and have offered detailed insights into the possible nature of intuition and its relationship to complex skilled performance, expert clinical judgement and the art of nursing. Returning to our example, the nurse would be able to draw upon empirical knowledge of common reactions of patients with cancer who are faced with poor prognoses and difficult decisions regarding treatment options, it is also likely that her personal experience of similar situations can be drawn upon and that her understanding of ethical theory will provide clarification about possible courses of action. In addition her personal knowledge will be a factor in recognising the situation which faces the patient as a fellow human being. Aesthetic knowing it is argued, will allow the nurse to respond immediately to the patients refusal to accept further treatment at that particular instant or moment, without apparent conscious deliberation about the alternatives. It is suggested that the nurse's ability to engage with the patient at this moment will lead to her intuiting a course of action which may include remaining quietly with the patient and seeking his permission to try and help the nurse to understand the reasons for his decision. The 'artistry' in this action is in the creative response to the unique situation for this particular patient at this point in time. The nurse demonstrates her genuine concern to understand this patient's situation as he sees it and to do this *before* she responds directly to his refusal of further treatment.

In listing the forms of knowledge identified by Carper (1978) it is important to point out that there is no intention to place the forms of knowing in a hierarchical order. It is believed that one form of knowledge should not be regarded as superior or inferior to another, but rather that each different form of knowledge is important in its own right and will be useful for some purpose. For nurses working in cancer and palliative care it is considered that provision of effective and appropriate care for individuals, families or groups will require integration of knowledge from all four forms and not simply a reliance on one form or another. Carper (1992) has further clarified her work on the fundamental patterns of knowing. There have been adaptations and development of the work (Johns, 1995; Heath, 1998). In addition there has been critical examination of the concepts of nursing art and aesthetics (Edwards, 1998, 2001; de Raeve, 1998). Despite some concerns about the comprehensiveness and validity of Carper's (1978) claims, the fundamental patterns of knowing remain influential in determination of curriculum content in nursing programmes, and also in the debate surrounding what constitutes appropriate knowledge for nursing. Carper's work, while originating in 1978, was not widely considered in the United Kingdom until the late 1980s, but it reflects a different type of 'nursing theory' to the narrow conception of nursing models as nursing theory. In the past ten years there has been a slow but recognisable shift in the nursing literature and in published work relating to theory in nursing. This shift has begun to focus on issues of considerable interest to cancer and palliative care nurses. Issues that now sit alongside pathophysiology and pharmacology in programmes of education, include quality of life, survivorship, the experience of fatigue and the concept of hope. These are issues that have been examined by nurse researchers and about which (nursing) theory has been developed. These issues are examples of nursing theory which can describe, explain and predict the ways in which some patients will respond to the diagnosis of cancer or the experience of chronic and disabling illness. This then is theory which has utility for practice.

Why Do We Need Theory in General and Nursing Theory in Particular?

People naturally seek to understand their world, indeed it is common to hear people say 'my theory about that event is...'. As we develop knowledge we seek understanding of how the different facts, ideas and experiences we are exposed to are related and can be explained in meaningful ways. Knowledge and theory are clearly linked in that the development of knowledge is based on identification, examination and explanation of concepts. For example, the concepts of denial and bargaining (Kubler-Ross, 1970) are important in the understanding of individual reactions to loss and grief. Theorists explore or test the relationships between concepts to arrive at descriptions or explanations of particular events, situations, or interactions. Theories aid in understanding events, behaviours, responses and experiences. Empirical theories can result in general laws, for example about the effects of gravitational force on the earth or about the behaviour of particular molecules when subjected to heating or cooling. These theories allow scientists in disciplines such as chemistry and physics to predict and control specific events or phenomena with complete accuracy. However, nursing as a discipline works with complex human beings and their individual reactions to health and illness, therefore theories developed about human responses will not result in generalised laws but in more tentative descriptions and explanations of phenomena, which can contribute to understanding, predicting and responding to human behaviour in health and illness.

Many definitions of theory are offered; some tend to reflect an emphasis on traditional scientific approaches, while others emphasise a more tentative and qualitative explanation of reality. Riehl and Roy (1980) suggested that theory was 'a logically interconnected set of propositions used to describe explain and predict a part of the empirical world' (p.7). This is a good example of a traditional 'scientific' definition of theory. More recently, Chinn and Kramer suggested that theory is 'a creative and rigorous structuring of ideas that project a tentative, purposeful and systematic view of phenomena' (1995, p.72). This second definition retains the emphasis on rigorous and systematic structuring of ideas but it acknowledges that the theory can be tentative, its purpose being to describe and explain rather than predict and control. The purpose of theory is another important consideration. Hunink (1995) points out that 'theories are means to achieve an end, rather than an end in themselves' (p.31). Also there is the view that the purpose of theory is to (help us) understand and illuminate the world (Watson, 1985). It is important to accept too that in helping us understand the world or elements within it, that theories are systematic abstractions of reality and are not the reality in itself (Chinn and Kramer, 1995). This may help define what a theory is, but it does not answer the question about why nursing needs theory. Most nurses today would accept that nursing practice or the provision of nursing care should be based on evidence of the efficacy of that care. Indeed the drive for evidence-based care (Muir-Gray, 1997; Closs and Cheater, 1999; French, 1999) and the clinical effectiveness agenda (NHSE, 1996) is based firmly on these principles. These are major factors affecting the work of advanced practitioners in cancer and palliative care. Theory in general and nursing theory in particular can make an important contribution to nurses' ability to provide evidence-based care; this will however depend on how well the theory is able to describe, explain, predict or control a part of the empirical world. Or if we take the Chinn and Kramer (1995) view, the measure of the value of the theory for practice will be the ability of the theory to tentatively, purposefully and usefully explain a part of reality for the patient and nurse. Some of the more general theories which have been accepted and used by nurses are theories of loss and grief (Kubler-Ross, 1970; Worden, 1983), theories relating to health beliefs (Becker, 1974) and theories of health behaviour and action (Prochaska *et al.*, 1992). It is important to point out that none of these theories has been regarded as complete or without flaws, each has been subject to challenge and revision over time. Nonetheless the theories might be said to have made a useful contribution to nursing practice in the past twenty years. Most disciplines accept, almost without question, that theories will be proposed, developed, tested and refined or rejected, this is the dynamic way in which knowledge and understanding of the world develops.

Several classification systems for theory have been developed. These focus on for example the purpose and levels of theory (Dickoff and James, 1968b; Stevens-Barnum, 1998), the type of theory and level of abstraction (Merton, 1968; Walker and Avant, 1995) and the theoretical derivation (Leddy and Pepper, 1998). Two of these classifications (Walker and Avant, 1995; Dickoff and James, 1968b) will be useful for the discussion here. James Dickoff and Patricia James are philosophers who were working at Yale University in the 1960s and had been working with nursing faculty and students on the nature of conceptual and theoretical issues in nursing. As a direct result of their interactions with nurses, Dickoff and James developed a seminal paper entitled 'a theory of theories: a position paper' in which they argued that nursing as a practice discipline must have an action orientation to theory development that aims ultimately to shape the reality of practice. Theory in a practice discipline according to Dickoff and James (1968a) must do more than describe in order to develop understanding, it must be able to predict and produce the desired reality. By this they meant that theory in nursing must be able to explain or predict the relationship between variables, in order that the highest level of theory, situation producing theory could be developed. Situation producing theory would provide prescriptions for action on the part of the practitioner to bring about desired goals. Dickoff and James (1968b) suggested four levels of theory (see below) and argued that nursing must develop situation producing (or prescriptive) theories which were generated from the development of theories at the lower levels. The usefulness of this classification will be considered in the next section.

The four levels of theory suggested by (Dickoff and James (1968b), are:

Level 1   Factor-isolating (naming) theories

Level 2   Factor-relating (situation depicting theories)

Level 3   Situation-relating theories
          (a) predictive theories
          (b) promoting or inhibiting theories

Level 4   Situation-producing (prescriptive) theories.

Walker and Avant (1995) provided a further useful framework for considering nursing theory. Four types are described; these are:

- Meta-theory;

- Grand theory;

- Middle-range theory;

- Practice theory.

Meta-theory can be regarded as theory about the nature of theory, and the philosophical processes for theory development. Dickoff and James's (1968a, 1968b) seminal work falls into this category, and the work of Meleis (1997), Walker and Avant (1995) and Fawcett (1995) may also be regarded as meta-theorising. This important activity, while not the interest or remit of everyone, effectively responds to Visitainer's (1986) challenge to clarify what knowledge is needed for nursing and to specify how that knowledge should be developed. Debate about the nature of knowledge needed for nursing and the development of theory has not always been highly valued in a practice discipline which is so closely aligned with a doing culture. However, these debates continue to challenge the discipline to clarify its areas of concern and how these can be investigated and articulated.

Grand theory includes broad, highly abstract and often global perspectives on existing ideas. Grand theories would aim to describe the whole of a phenomenon rather than a distinct part of it. Most nursing models can be regarded as grand theories in that at their current stage of development, they contain vague terminology and have not clearly articulated the relationship between concepts identified (Walker and Avant, 1995; McKenna, 1997). Grand theories cannot be tested empirically (Fawcett, 1995) but have made a contribution to the discipline in that they have focused attention on describing and explaining the distinctive nursing contribution in healthcare, and on the roles that nurses can develop in provision of effective care. While grand theories cannot in themselves be empirically tested, some of the concepts that have been developed by these theorists have been subject to empirical testing. For example, the concept of self care derives from Orem's (1970, 1995) 'Self Care Deficit Theory of Nursing' and has been subject to empirical investigation by Kubricht (1984), Woods (1985) and Taylor (1990). The high level of abstraction of these theories and their attempts to describe and explain the whole of nursing are both contributory factors leading to the frustration which many nurses have experienced in trying to apply the theories to their practice. There is growing recognition that the development of grand theory reflects an important stage in the development of theory in nursing, but that theory at the grand level mainly represents attempts to delineate the areas of knowledge and practice which are claimed to be the primary concern of nurses. Rather than an end point in the development of a knowledge base for the discipline, grand theories represent a stage in the theoretical development of the discipline. These theories can be said in most cases to constitute theory at levels 1 and 2 in the Dickoff and James (1968a) classification.

In recent years there has been increasing interest in the development of middle range theory both in the United States and in the United Kingdom (McKenna, 1997; Lenz, 1998; Liehr and Smith, 1999). The term middle range theory was first coined by the sociologist Robert Merton (1968). Theory at the middle range level is characterised by a concentration on a limited number of concepts and variables. The theories do not attempt to describe or explain the whole of the discipline, but rather specific elements of concern to the discipline. Middle range theories are claimed to guide research into practice, to generate testable hypotheses and to be more easily applicable in the practice setting. Middle range theories which could be important for advancing practice in cancer and palliative care nursing include the 'Chronic Illness Trajectory' framework (Corbin and Strauss, 1991), the 'Theory of Unpleasant Symptoms' (Lenz *et al.*, 1997) and the 'Balance between Analgesia and Side Effects' (Good and Moore, 1996). These theories have generally been developed inductively, that is, from observation and research in practice settings. The conceptual frameworks developed by these theorists demonstrate clear relationships between concepts; the components of the theory are explicit and intelligible to the reader. Classifying these theories according to their ability to describe, explain or predict situations, responses or actions, would place most of the theories in the predictive category (level 3). For example, the Theory of Unpleasant Symptoms is based on the assumption that 'there are sufficient commonalities among symptoms to warrant a theory that is not limited to one symptom, but can explain and guide research and practice regarding an array of unpleasant symptoms' (Lenz *et al.*, 1997, p.14). In proposing and explaining the (unpleasant) symptoms experienced by individuals, the factors that give rise to or affect the nature of the symptom experience, and the consequences (for the individual) of the symptom experience; it is possible to predict how unpleasant symptoms may affect the individual in the performance of his physical, cognitive and social activities. Merton (1968) suggested that middle-range theories were particularly important for practice disciplines, and there appears to be considerable contemporary support for this view in the nursing literature (Chinn, 1997; Lenz *et al.*, 1997; Liehr and Smith, 1999). It is important to point out here that development of middle-range theory will not replace or remove the need for theory at the grand level. The development of middle-range theory offers an opportunity for nursing practice and nursing scholarship to continue to develop the knowledge base of nursing on which good practice can be based.

The last level of theory in the framework described above is practice theory. Dickoff and James (1968b) identified situation-producing theory (prescriptive or practice theory) as the highest level of theory and the level at which a practice discipline such as nursing should aim. Practice theory is designed to provide nurses in practice with prescriptive guidelines or instructions for practice. For example, in the context of information provision to reduce anxiety; theory at the middle range may predict that if specific treatment intervention information is given using language with which the patient is familiar, and which covers common sources of anxiety, for example nature and duration of treatment, side effects, likelihood of pain and pain control, effect of treatment on disease process; then anxiety is likely to be reduced and compliance with advice is likely to be improved. At the practice theory level, this prediction would be developed into a specific intervention which would provide direction or guides for nursing action designed to bring about the desired goal of anxiety reduction. Thus in a situation where a specific chemotherapy regime is required, nurses may be directed to use a specific information or teaching package in pre-admission consultation. The patient would then go home with specific written information and a telephone contact number. The understanding of information would then be checked again at the time of admission and repeated if necessary. These interventions can be tested to determine the reduction in anxiety and improvement in treatment compliance and recovery brought about by the use of the intervention. Theory at the practice level is of real interest to practising nurses, particularly in the current climate, which demands that practice is based on sound evidence of its efficacy. The challenge for both practising nurses and nurse scholars is to continue to develop theory which has practical utility, is regarded as significant by the profession, and which can be tested empirically.

Going Beyond the Theory–Practice Gap

So far this chapter has argued that theory in nursing has an important contribution to make to the development of nursing practice in general, and practice in cancer and palliative care specifically. However, the chapter would not be complete without some consideration of the so called 'theory–practice gap'. This issue may well have been overstated in that, few if any theorists or practitioners, would deny that nursing practice and theory in nursing have always been in dynamic interaction as both have sought to advance the knowledge and practice of the discipline in order to provide the care required by those who need nursing. There are, however, several different opinions about the nature of the interaction between theory in nursing and nursing practice.

Some Positions in the Theory–Practice Gap Debate

It is not the purpose of this section of the chapter to deny the existence of a theory–practice gap. It will be argued however that by investing time and energy in seeking to lay the blame for the so-called gap at the of door of either theorists or practitioners, or indeed both of these groups, nursing runs the risk of becoming enmeshed in unproductive, unnecessary and at times adversarial debate which does little to develop the practice of nursing. The main positions in the theory–practice gap debate can be summarised as follows:

- Theorists and academics are to blame for the gap as the theories they develop or teach are too far removed from the realities of practice to be useful (Reed and Proctor, 1993; Rolfe, 1996; Upton, 1999);

- Nursing theory should be developed from practice by practitioners and then be tested and modified in that setting (Burrows and McLeish, 1995; Rolfe, 1996, 1997);

- The theory–practice gap is inevitable, necessary and desirable in that the dynamic tension that exists between theory and practice is the basis of change and development in the practice setting (Cook, 1991; Rafferty *et al.*, 1996; Walker, 1997).

A common feature of the first position is that academics, theorists and researchers have tended to hold the view that if theory or research findings are not implemented in practice then the fault is not that of the theory or research (Gibbings, 1993; NHSE, 1996). The fault or failure in this position is seen to be either the method of communicating the findings or of the practitioners in the clinical setting. It could be argued that this was the position adopted by those advocating the widespread adoption of nursing models (grand theories) in the 1980s and early 1990s. Rolfe (1996, 1997) argues that few academics or researchers have been willing to examine whether it is the inadequacy of the theories themselves, or the failure of academics and researchers to understand the realities of practice, which has maintained a theory–practice gap. There is some merit in this position if it moves from apportioning of blame to an honest appraisal of ways in which theory and practice can develop a reciprocal and beneficial relationship. That this is necessary is given even more urgency by the current professional and policy drivers for practice to be based on sound evidence of its efficacy (NHSE, 1996).

The second position is a response to the first in that it seeks to question the dominant position of traditional science in determining what counts as knowledge. It also seeks to challenge the power of leading academics and researchers in nursing who conduct research and publish their findings and views, to create and legitimise knowledge. Alternative approaches to knowledge are proposed by those who support this position. These approaches tend to focus on action research (Rolfe, 1996), reflective practice (Schon, 1983), and the concept of praxis (Benner, 1984; Reed, 1995; Rolfe, 1996; Thorne and Hayes, 1997). The term praxis in this context refers to the view that there can be unity between theory and practice or a coming together of theory and practice. This unity can be brought about by reflection on action, and development and testing of informal theory which is context specific. No claims are made for the ability of theory to cover all situations, rather there is an acceptance that the development of theory in this way will have immediate local relevance for the practitioner in the context of providing care for a specific individual. Theory in this case develops from, is modified by and directly influences practice (Rolfe, 1996). It is clear then that arguments for a theory–practice gap would be more difficult to sustain if the dominant approach to theory generation was the nursing praxis approach.

It is acknowledged, however, by some leading proponents of the nursing praxis approach, that a wholesale rejection of formal theory in favour of the adoption of an informal theory or nursing praxis paradigm, would not be adequate to represent the entire knowledge base on which nursing practice should be based (Paul and Heaslip, 1995; Benner *et al.*, 1996). Middle-range and practice theories have the potential to respond to the concerns which characterise this second position. The key issue for those who accept that nursing praxis alone will not provide all the knowledge needed for practice, is for the knowledge that is developed from middle-range or practice theories to provide description, explanation and perhaps prescriptions for nursing care and nursing interventions, which are relevant to the concerns or problems encountered by practising nurses in their everyday practice. In short, the purpose of theory generation must be to develop knowledge for practice in cancer and palliative care as opposed to academic advancement.

The third position in this debate is a pragmatic, but still contentious one. Some commentators such as Rafferty *et al.* (1996) and Walker (1997) hold the view that attempts to bring about a harmonisation of theory and practice are counter productive. It is argued that removing the dynamic tension that exists between theory and practice will be harmful to both, in that the political, social and professional contexts in which practice takes place and develops, will continue to demand more sophisticated knowledge and understanding of the nature of nursing practice. This in turn will demand of academics and theorists, a critical examination of practice concerns and the development of theoretical explanations which are both robust and relevant in the world or practice. Rolfe (1997) is critical of this position suggesting it may be misleading and potentially dangerous. Rolfe (1997) draws the analogy of a theory–practice gap in engineering and makes the point that such a gap would put lives at risk. This position is perhaps deliberately overstated as even in engineering, theoretical pluralism and diversity exists as theoretical models and explanations are developed, tested, and accepted or rejected before structures such as bridges or buildings are constructed. In summary, there is merit in all of these positions as explanations for factors underlying the theory–practice gap in nursing. The position taken in this chapter is, however, that while the debate will continue to stake the claims for one position as opposed to another, the main challenge facing practitioners, academics and theorists is to develop an openness to the contributions that different approaches to the generation, testing and application of knowledge in nursing. For nurses engaged in advancing practice in cancer and palliative care the issue will not be in seeking to prove the worthiness of one knowledge claim against another, but rather the issue will be about 'what is valid and reliable' in improving the care of patients.

Conclusion

This chapter has attempted to focus on the relationship that nurses have had with theory in nursing, which has been at times indifferent or intolerant. Some of the reasons for this problematic relationship, in terms of the abstract nature and level of some of the information which became known as nursing models and nursing theories, were explored, and it was suggested that this was a too narrow and restricted conception of theory in nursing. A broader discussion on the nature of knowledge needed in nursing suggested that a position first advocated by Carper in 1978, that nursing knowledge cannot be aligned with only one paradigm or perspective, was more useful. The theory–practice gap debate, it was argued, may sharpen our understanding of the issues which affect both practitioners and theorists but at the end of the day it can only be useful if it enables nurses to move beyond the debate and onto the practical reality of developing knowledge which leads to better care for patients. Nursing's challenge is not simply to pick up that which is useful from the many perspectives available, be they traditional scientific, interpretive or indeed postmodern in origin. The challenge is to critically examine the knowledge from these perspectives in the context of the specific practice concerns which affect the daily provision of care to patients and their relatives, and to synthesise and disseminate this 'nursing knowledge' in order to develop and advance that care.

References

Becker, M.H. (ed.) (1974) *The Health Belief Model and Personal Health Behaviour*. New Jersey: Slack.

Benner, P. (1984) *From Novice to Expert: excellence and power in clinical nursing practice*. Menlo Park, CA: Addison-Wesley.

Benner, P. and C. Tanner (1987) How expert nurses use intuition. *American Journal of Nursing*, 87, 23–31.

Benner, P., C. Tanner and C. Chesla (1996) *Expertise in nursing practice: Caring clinical judgement and ethics*. New York: Springer.

Bond, M. (1986) *Stress and Self Awareness: A guide for nurses*. London: Heinemann.

Burnard, P. (1985) *Learning Human Skills*. London: Heinemann.

Burrows, D. and K. McLeish (1995) A model for research based practice. *Journal of Clinical Nursing*, 4, 243–7.

Carper, B.A. (1978) Fundamental patterns of knowing in nursing. *Advances in Nursing Science*, Oct., 1(1), 13–23.

Carper, B.A. (1992) Philosophical Enquiry in nursing: an application in J.F. Kikuchi and H. Simmons (eds) (1992) *Philosophical Enquiry in Nursing*. Newbury Park: Sage.

Chenoweth, L. (1998) Facilitating the process of critical thinking for nursing. *Nurse Education Today*, 18, 281–92.

Chinn, P.L. (1997) Why Middle Range Theory? Editorial. *Advances in Nursing Science*, 19(3), viii.

Chinn, P.L. and M.K. Kramer (1995) *Theory and Nursing: A systematic approach*. 4th edn St Louis: Mosby.

Clarke, D.J. and J. Holt (2001) Philosophy: A key to open the door to critical thinking. *Nurse Education Today*, 21, 71–8.

Closs, S.J. and F.M. Cheater (1999) Evidence for nursing practice: a clarification of the issues. *Journal of Advanced Nursing*, 30(1), 10–17.

Cody, W.K (1996) Drowning in eclecticism. *Nursing Science Quarterly*, 9, 86–8.

Concise Oxford Dictionary (1990) 8th edn. Oxford: Clarendon Press.

Cook, S. (1991) Mind the theory-practice gap in nursing. *Journal of Advanced Nursing*, 16, 1462–9.

Corbin, J.M. and A. Strauss (1991) A nursing model for chronic illness management based upon the trajectory framework. *Scholarly Enquiry for Nursing Practice: An International Journal*. 5(3), 155–74.

de Raeve, L. (1998) The Art of Nursing: An aesthetics? *Nursing Ethics*, 5(5), 401–11.

Department of Health (1999) *Making a Difference: Strengthening the nursing, midwifery and health visiting contribution to health and healthcare*. London: Department of Health.

Dickoff, J. and P. James (1968a) A theory of theories: A position paper. *Nursing Research*, May–June, 17(3), 197–203.

Dickoff, J. and P. James (1968b) Theory in practice discipline part 1: Practice oriented theory. *Nursing Research*, September–October, 17(5), 415–35.

Donaldson, S. and D. Crowley (1978) The discipline of nursing. *Nursing Outlook*, 26, 113–20.

Edwards, S.D. (1998) The Art of Nursing. *Nursing Ethics*, 5(5), 393–400.

Edwards, S.D. (2001) *Philosophy of Nursing: An Introduction*. Basingstoke: Palgrave – now Palgrave Macmillan.

Emden, C. (1991) Ways of knowing in nursing, in G. Gray and R. Pratt (eds), *Towards a Discipline of Nursing*. Edinburgh: Churchill Livingstone.

Fawcett, J. (1995) *Analysis and Evaluation of Theories of Nursing*. 3rd edn. Philadelphia: F.A. Davis.

French, P. (1999) The development of evidence based nursing. *Journal of Advanced Nursing*, 29(1), 72–8.

Freire, P. (1972) *Cultural action for freedom*. Harmondsworth: Penguin.

Gibbings, S. (1993) Informed Action. *Nursing Times*, 89(46), 28–31.

Glen, S. (1995) Developing critical thinking in higher education. *Nurse Education Today*, 15(3), 170–76.

Good, M. and S.M. Moore (1996) Clinical Practice Guidelines as a new source of middle range theory: focus on acute pain. *Nursing Outlook*, 44, 74–9.

Heath, H. (1998) Reflection and patterns of knowing in nursing. *Journal of Advanced Nursing*, 27(5), 1054–9.

Henderson, V. (1966) *The Nature of Nursing: a definition and its implications for practice, education and research*. London: Collier Macmillan.

Hunink, G. (1995) *A Study Guide to Nursing Theories*. Edinburgh: Campion Press.

Johns, C. (ed.) (1994) *The Burford NDU Model: Caring in Practice*. Oxford: Blackwell Scientific.

Johns, C. (1995) Framing learning through reflection within Carper's fundamental ways of knowing in nursing. *Journal of Advanced Nursing*, 22(2), 226–34.

Kubler-Ross, E. (1970) *On death and dying*. London: Tavistock.

Kubricht, D.W. (1984) Therapeutic Self Care Demands expressed by outpatients receiving external radiation therapy. *Cancer Nursing*, 7, 43–52.

Leddy, S. and J.M. Pepper (1998) *Conceptual Bases of Professional Nursing*. 4th edn. Philadelphia: Lippincott.

Lenz, E.R. (1998) Role of Middle Range Theory for Nursing Research and Practice: Part 1 Nursing Research. *Nursing Leadership Forum*, 3(1), Spring, 24–33.

Lenz, E.R., L.C. Pugh, R.A. Milligan, A. Gift and F. Suppe (1997) The Middle Range Theory of Unpleasant Symptoms: An update. *Advances in Nursing Science*, 19(3), 14–27.

Liehr, P. and M.J. Smith (1999) Middle Range Theory: Spinning research and practice to create knowledge for the new millennium. *Advances in Nursing Science*, 21(4), 81–91.

Macleod-Clark, J. (1984) Communication: the continuing challenge. *Nursing Times*, 84(23), 24–7.

Manley, K. (1997) Knowledge for nursing practice in A. Perry (ed) *Nursing: A knowledge base for practice*. 2nd edn. London: Arnold.

McKenna, H. (1997) *Nursing Theories and Models*. London: Routledge.

McMahon, R. and A. Pearson (1995) *Nursing as Therapy*. Chapman Hall: London.

Meleis, A.I. (1997) *Theoretical Nursing: Development and Progress*. 3rd edn. Philadelphia: Lippincott.

Merton, R.K. (1968) *Social Theory and Social Structure*. New York: Free Press.

Muir-Gray, J.A. (1997) *Evidence Based Healthcare. How to make health policy and management decisions*. Edinburgh: Churchill Livingstone.

Neeson, B., A. Faulkner and J. Macleod-Clark (1984) Teaching Communication Skills: Evaluation of the development of communication skills. Part 2. *Nurse Education Today*, (4)3, 54–7.

Neuman, B. (1982) *The Neuman Systems Model: Application to nursing education and practice*. Norwalk, CT: Appleton and Lange.

NHS Executive (1996) *Promoting Clinical Effectiveness: A framework for action in and through the NHS. A position statement*. Department of Health: Leeds.

Orem, D.E. (1970) *Nursing: Concepts of Practice*. New York: McGraw-Hill.

Orem, D.E. (1995) *Nursing: Concepts of Practice*. 5th edn. New York: McGraw-Hill.

Paul, R.W. and P. Heaslip (1995) Critical thinking and intuitive practice in nursing. *Journal of Advanced Nursing*, 22, 40–47.

Pearson, A. (1992) *Nursing at Burford: A story of change*. London: Scutari Press.

Peplau, H.E. (1952) *Interpersonal Relations in Nursing*. New York: Puttnam.

Peplau, H.E. (1988) *Interpersonal Relations in Nursing*. (Reprinted) New York: Puttnam.

Prochaska, J.O., C. DiClemente and J.C. Norcross (1992) In search of how people change: applications to addictive behaviours. *American Psychologist*, 47, 1102–14.

Rafferty, A.M., N. Allcock and J. Lathlean (1996) The theory–practice 'gap': taking issue with the issue. *Journal of Advanced Nursing*, 23, 685–91.

Rafferty, A.M. (1998) *The politics of nursing knowledge*. London: Routledge.

Reed, J. (1995) Using a group project to teach research methods. *Nurse Education Today*, 15(1), 56–60.

Reed, J. and S. Proctor (1993) *Nurse education: A reflective approach*. London: Edward Arnold.

Riehl, J.P. and C. Roy (1980) *Conceptual Models for Nursing Practice*. 2nd edn. New York: Appleton Century Crofts.

Rogers, C. (1983) *Freedom to Learn for the 80's*. Ohio: Merrill.

Rolfe, G. (1996) *Closing the theory practice gap: a new paradigm for nursing*. Oxford: Butterworth-Heinemann.

Rolfe, G. (1997) Nursing Praxis: a zealot responds. Janforum. *Journal of Advanced Nursing*, 25, 426–7.

Roy, C. (1984) *Introduction to nursing: An Adaptation Model*. 2nd edn. Englewood Cliffs, NJ: Prentice-Hall.

Schön, D.A. (1983) *The reflective practitioner: how professionals think in action*. New York: Basic Books.

Stevens-Barnum, B. (1998) *Nursing Theory: Analysis, application, evaluation*. 5th edn. New York: Lippincott.

Taylor, S.G. (1990) Self Care Deficit Theory and Research, in C. Metzger-McQuiston and A.A. Webb (eds) (1995) *Foundations of Nursing Theory*. London: Sage.

Thorne, S.A. and V.E. Hayes (eds) (1997) *Nursing Praxis: Knowledge and action*. London: Sage.

UKCC (1986) *Project 2000; A new preparation to practice*. London: UKCC.

Upton. D. (1999) How can we have evidence-based practice if we have a theory-practice gap in nursing today? *Journal of Advanced Nursing*, 29(3), 549–55.

Visitainer, M. (1986) The nature of knowledge and theory in nursing. *Image*, 18, 32–8.

Walker, K. (1997) Dangerous liaisons: thinking, doing, nursing. *Collegian*, 4(2), April, 4–14.

Walker, L.O. and K.C. Avant (1995) *Strategies for Theory Construction in Nursing*. 3rd edn. Norwalk, CT: Appleton and Lange.

Watson, J. (1985) *Nursing: Human Science and Human Care*. New York: Appleton Century Crofts.

Woods, N.F. (1985) Self care practices among young adult married women. *Research in Nursing and Health*, 8, 21–31.

Worden, J.W. (1983) *Grief Counselling and Grief Therapy*. London: Tavistock.

Wright, S.G. (1986) *Building and Using a Model of Nursing*. London: Edward Arnold.

4

Advancing Practice Through Research

SUSAN HOLMES

When we, as individual practitioners, provide care to individual patients, we do this on the basis of our knowledge and previous experience; as we gain increased knowledge and/or experience the way in which that care is provided may be modified – as, indeed, it should be. While this is undoubtedly the case, and results in enhanced patient care, it also raises many questions such as how we decide what to do in individual cases or why we vary the care delivered to different patients experiencing the same (or similar) symptoms or suffering from the same condition. Do we use 'traditional' methods of care 'handed down' to us by those who have gone before? Do we base our approach on 'trial and error' or do we truly make our decisions on the basis of knowledge gleaned from scientific enquiry? In other words, do we use evidence to underpin our care delivery or take active steps to 'advance' (or change) practice? It can be argued that the focus of an advanced practitioner is to do just that.

Indeed, the thesis inherent in this text is that advanced practitioners are those who are able to both recognise and challenge the assumptions underlying nursing practice, to identify and articulate the nursing role and its contribution to healthcare and, ultimately, to the outcome for patients. To achieve this necessarily requires skills in both clinical decision-making and professional judgement which, in turn, require the synthesis of personal, experiential and scientific knowledge (Clark *et al.*, 1996). This combination is, of course, designed both to promote and develop practice through the provision of clinical leadership (Holmes, 1991) and to enhance the care received by patients regardless of the nature of their primary disease.

To achieve this successfully requires that nursing in general, and advanced practice in particular, are redefined 'beyond the modern industrial production line view toward a more mature professional practice' (Watson, 1998). In other words, since nursing clearly holds a central role in the constantly changing and increasingly complex healthcare environment, it must re-evaluate and clearly delineate its role and, perhaps more importantly, differentiate between the nursing model and the medical model enabling it to demonstrate its unique contribution to healthcare (Spitzer, 1998). By promoting care that truly takes account of individual needs, while acknowledging the patient's medical condition and focusing on clearly demonstrable outcomes, nursing is a process that is carried out in the context of the specific relationship developed between nurse and patient (Rolfe, 1998). Ensuring that this is founded on a sound theoretical base and underpinned by the development of a true nursing science, will help nursing to emerge as a healthcare discipline in its own right. This is vital within the current healthcare environment, with its emphasis on 'evidence' and 'outcomes', when nursing must be in a position to develop its practice in ways that enable it to clearly demonstrate both its efficacy and its effectiveness almost regardless of the medical diagnosis or treatment. In other words, nursing (and nurses) must be able to explicate its role as a therapeutic entity in its own right separate from, but complementary to, the roles of other healthcare practitioners. The need to identify the role of nurses, and differentiate this from other healthcare roles, is also important in increasing the accountability of the profession to patients for the nursing component of their care (Bond and Thomas, 1991). Although the role of the advanced practitioners is crucial in this regard, none of this will be possible without critical evaluation and research.

Thus, while the advanced practitioner must be seen to ground their practice in everyday reality they must, simultaneously, point the way towards establishing evidence-based outcomes that serve to demonstrate the essential aspects of nursing and, concurrently, ensure the best possible delivery of patient care and enhanced patient outcome. In this way, advanced clinical practice will be seen to be moving the thinking about nursing forward in a way that causes it to examine and re-examine its underlying tenets, to shift away from its previous reliance on 'myth, tradition and anecdote' (Walsh and Ford, 1992; Maynard, 1994) towards making greater use of science, research and evidence to guide practice (Appleby *et al.*, 1995).

Advancing practice thus forces nurses to rethink their common behaviours and practices bringing new knowledge to the fore while sifting the old retaining its strengths and disposing of its weaknesses. It also forces a reconceptualisation of nursing itself allowing its complexities to be explored and, in this way, distinguishing it from other healthcare disciplines thus enhancing its value. Such an approach will enable new 'traditions' to be developed, on the basis of a sound theoretical and scientific foundation that will advance both nursing practice and research; it will provide the foundation on which to build by transforming the 'old' skills and knowledge into a soundly based nursing science to underpin the care delivered to all patients. The advanced practitioner is ideally placed to play a central role in such activity.

The Evidence-Based Culture

Recent National Health Service (NHS) reforms, together with the research and development (R&D) strategy (Department of Health (DoH), 1991; 1993a; 2001), place the emphasis firmly upon the need for healthcare provision to be 'evidence-based' and to be shown to be both efficient and effective (Gray, 1997). This has been supported by the development of a strategy for research in nursing, midwifery and health visiting (DoH, 1993b; 2001). Education, training, funding for research and the integration of research and development with practice were also addressed the objective being to enhance the research skills and training received by practitioners and to ensure that research in nursing was firmly located within the broader context of health services research (DoH, 1993b). It is, however, also recognised that not all nurses can or should themselves undertake research and that a minority is likely to pursue a research career; all practitioners are, however, required to use research – and evidence derived from research – to inform and underpin their practice (DoH, 1993b; Hardey and Mulhall, 1994). This means that nurses, like all healthcare practitioners, are increasingly required to justify and account for their actions in terms of their efficacy, effectiveness and, increasingly, cost.

It is easy to believe that this is a new approach but this is not, in fact, the case and the concept of research-based practice was first introduced by the Briggs Committee on Nursing (Department of Health and Social Security (DHSS), 1972) which recommended that nursing should develop into a research-based profession while McFarlane (1980) emphasised the need to direct nursing care appropriately and to increase its scientific basis. Nurses in general have been slow to accept these challenges and there is little evidence to suggest that these recommendations have been adopted by the profession as a whole (McSherry, 1997) or even that the application of nursing theories, designed to provide a rationale for planning care intended to meet individual needs, has contributed to the development of a body of knowledge about either clinical interventions and/or the outcomes of nursing care (Schober, 1995).

Indeed, it is claimed that many, if not the majority of procedures to which patients are exposed by healthcare practitioners have little, if any, scientific basis (Maynard, 1994). Similarly, Blumenthal (1994) reveals that many patients receive different treatment(s) even when suffering the same clinical condition. It is variations such as these, combined with the almost inevitable variability in effectiveness, that demonstrate one of

Figure 4.1   Implementation of evidence-based practice

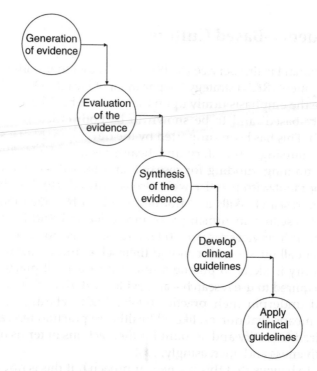

Source: Rosenberg and Donald (1995).

the major driving forces underlying the move towards evidence-based practice a concept defined as 'an approach to problem solving in clinical practice' (Rosenberg and Donald, 1995). This, therefore, involves identifying the clinical problem, searching the literature, critically evaluating the evidence and, finally, determining the intervention(s) on the basis of demonstrable effectiveness and/or efficiency (See Figure 4.1). In other words, today's healthcare requires that all interventions and professional judgements are substantiated (Rolfe, 1998).

The 'evidence-based culture' thus offers nurses – and particularly the advanced practitioner – the opportunity both to develop their skills and to demonstrate their efficacy in determining patient outcome (Thompson, 1998a). This, accompanied by the increasing involvement of patients (consumers/users/clients), although not new to either cancer or palliative care, increases the accountability of nurses to their patients and, in turn, requires that decisions regarding care are justified on the basis of their known efficacy and effectiveness. Care provision is, therefore, increasingly exposed to scrutiny from a wide variety of sources including from nurses themselves. The advanced practitioner should be at the forefront of such developments helping to demonstrate the contribution made by nurses to patient outcome.

Evidence-Based Practice (EBP)

EBP appears to reflect the 'simple' drive for cost containment and value for money within the health service with the effect that 'effectiveness' and 'efficiency' have become the central goals of healthcare. The assumption is that achieving these goals will have a profound impact on clinical activities resulting in 'better' care for patients and, necessarily, achieving health improvements; it is also assumed that EBP will substantially reduce expenditure on ineffective or unproven diagnostic or therapeutic procedures (Appleby *et al.*, 1995). However, although Peckham (1991) believed firmly in the need for research-based healthcare, others have argued that the use of research, and/or its influence on health policy, has been minimal, 'so rare as to be negligible' (Hunter and Polit, 1992). In any case, effectiveness and efficiency (defined as desired outcome and value for money) may not, alone, be appropriate indicators of EBP; in combination they may be more powerful provided that the costs considered include not only the financial and the time of healthcare practitioners but also the human costs (to patients) and the 'appropriateness' of particular interventions for use in specific conditions or patient/client groups. Thus assessment of the evidence underlying practice may, at its simplest, reflect practice that is based on accurate and relevant information and, at its most complex, represent practice that is based on knowledge derived not only from research but also from nursing theory and clinical knowledge encompassing both life events and nursing experience (le May *et al.*, 1998). In other words, practice which reflects the view of Sackett *et al.* (1996) who define evidence-based medicine as: 'the conscientious and judicious use of current best evidence in making decisions about the care of individual patients' and expect that individual clinical experience will be integrated with that 'best evidence' to achieve optimal care (see Table 4.1).

This approach, in fact, enhances the 'tradition' inherent in healthcare, of taking an eclectic approach to the generation of evidence ranging from the scientific or humanistic to personal experience (Clarke, 1999) enabling nursing to 'borrow' evidence from other disciplines to inform its practice.

Sackett *et al.* (1996) highlight the importance of both evidence and clinical expertise considering both to be important. They state: 'Without clinical expertise, practice risks becoming tyrannized by evidence but

Table 4.1   Benefits of evidence-based practice

For patients	Reduced time wasted on inappropriate treatments
	Enhanced consistency in care
	Increased understanding of both investigations and treatment
	Increased confidence in practitioners and the NHS as a whole
For clinical practitioners	Active involvement in determining the appropriateness and effectiveness of care
	Redefining and/or changing practice in accordance with evidence where this is necessary
	Using clinical audit to enhance the quality of care
	Collecting/presenting evidence of the benefits of practice to patients and carers
	Increased accountability for care provisions
For the NHS as a whole	Enabling consistent decision-making
	Reducing variation in services
	Promoting cost-effectiveness
	Integration of activities (e.g. research and development, clinical audit, continuing professional development)
	Increasing accountability to the public for the service provided

Source: From le May (1999).

without best available evidence practice risks becoming rapidly out of date' (p. 71).

This should be of comfort to practitioners since their skills are recognised and, indeed, practitioners' views about the use of evidence emphasise its potential value in guiding practice (see Table 4.2). This does not, however, obviate the need to ensure that all clinical practice is founded on up-to-date information and research findings (DoH, 1989). Evidence-based healthcare, and advancing practice are, therefore, about integrating research with clinical expertise (Thompson, 1998b) (see Figure 4.2).

On the Nature of Evidence

The preceding section reveals why the phrase 'evidence-based' is increasingly entering the rhetoric of healthcare in general and nursing in particular. Similarly, it stresses the need for evidence on which to base healthcare interventions. This, in turn, necessitates consideration of the nature of that evidence and the way in which such evidence is obtained. Although there is

Table 4.2 Practitioners' views of evidence-based practice

Evidence based practice will help to:

- Demonstrate effectiveness
- Improve care
- Justify skill mix
- Solve problems
- Identify needs
- Provide a rationale for practice
- Provide consistent information
- Enhance professional status
- Show purchasers the value of evidence-based practice.

Source: Foundation of Nursing Studies (1996).

no doubt that evidence from any source can be helpful in attempts to advance practice and to enhance patient care there is, in reality, a 'hierarchy of evidence' (see Table 4.3) at the top of which is experimental research and the randomised controlled trial (RCT) and, at the bottom, the knowledge gained from experience (experiential knowledge) (White, 1997). Although this appears to devalue the role of experience, it is clear that Sackett *et al.* (1996) and others value both 'best evidence' and clinical experience equally; practitioners would, no doubt, argue that, if practice is to be enhanced, a combination of evidence and professional judgement is essential.

This, however, moves us little further forward since the nature of that evidence requires elucidation as Clarke (1999) stresses in challenging the belief that EBP emphasises the value of one type of evidence – that of experimental research and the RCT. French (1999) suggests that this reflects

Table 4.3 The 'hierarchy' of evidence

1. Evidence from randomised controlled trials
2. Evidence from controlled trials (without randomisation)
3. Evidence from case-controlled or cohort studies
4. Evidence from comparisons between times or places with or without intervention
5. Opinions from respected authorities (based on clinical experience), descriptive studies, or reports of expert committees.

Source: From Long (1996).

Figure 4.2   Integrating research with clinical practice

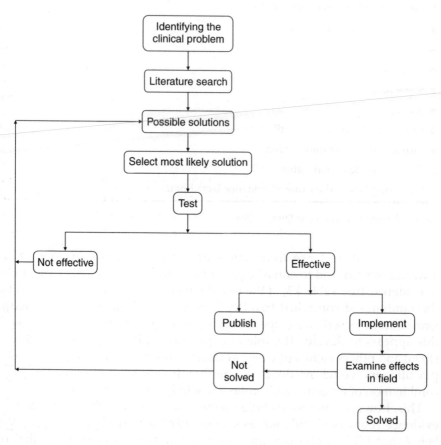

Source: Thompson (1998b).

the derivation of EBP which, in being derived from the concept of evidence-based *medicine*, medicalises the healthcare environment thus overlooking possible contributions from other scientific perspectives thereby creating as many problems as it solves. Certainly human beings (as are our patients) are a complex amalgam of the biological, the social and the psychological and exposed to influences from a wide variety of sources. To overlook these, and to value only the positivist (experimental) perspective on evidence, disregards the qualitative and humanistic aspects (French, 1999) and does a great disservice to our patients/clients. It also suggests that interpretative or qualitative research is associated with a lack of scientific rigour largely because such data rarely have global validity and so cannot be generalised beyond the population studied (Berragan, 1998); it may, however, enhance understanding of particular clinical problems or client groups and, through this, advance clinical practice in specific areas.

By overlooking the context in which care is delivered and the particular client group under consideration, the omission of qualitative evidence may damage nursing and the development of nursing practice. To confine 'evidence' only to that generated through RCTs aligns evidence-based practice with the medical model (French, 1999) and overlooks psycho-social and environmental aspects of health and illness and the care required. Lorentzon (1995) asserts that, in aligning themselves firmly with the medical model, nurses would fail to acknowledge the mixture of 'art and science' that is nursing. Despite this, many believe that qualitative research is unscientific and anecdotal. However, as many practitioners are quick to point out, practice is more than the 'simple' application of scientific rules (Naylor, 1995) so that knowledge that values not only science but also the subjective nature of human beings enables us to develop evidence that is realistic and useful for practice (Schumacher and Gortner, 1992). It is for this reason that findings from qualitative work are now increasingly accepted (DiCenso *et al.*, 1998).

The relationship between nursing and scientific knowledge must not, however, be underestimated. The natural sciences have and will continue to provide useful information (Berragan, 1998); from this, practice will advance. Biomedical knowledge will continue to provide the underpinning of much of the nursing role (Gould, 1999). Evidence for nursing can, there-fore, be derived from a variety of sources each of which has a particular place in the generation of knowledge (see Table 4.4). To generate effective evidence designed to advance practice and raise the quality of patient care the need for pluralism in approaches has never been more clear. This is essential if nurses and nursing are to ensure that the full range of the complexities underlying nursing and nursing care become visible to the world at large (Traynor and Rafferty, 1997).

The Research Imperative

As can be seen, research provides one means through which evidence to guide practice can be generated yet, to date, there is little 'evidence' to support claims that nursing is a research-based profession (Stevens, 1997). Indeed, Luker and Kenrick (1995) report that many practitioners fail to recognise that research has any relevance to their daily work and so seek no role for themselves in developing practice through research. Moreover, Closs and Cheater (1994), among many others, report that practice remains heavily influenced by strong personal beliefs founded on a combination of

Table 4.4   Sources of evidence for nursing practice

Source	Accessing
Evidence from research	Involves searching published and unpublished literature – original; (primary) research, literature reviews (secondary sources), clinical guidelines, published research-based standards of care
Evidence based on experience (professional or general)	Reflecting on practice – articulating reflections, facilitating discussion and searching the literature
Experience based on theory (not research-based)	Involves searching the literature (published or unpublished), learning from others and facilitating discussions
Evidence gathered from patients and/or their carers	Searching the literature for experiential writings and/or research findings, using audit data, analysing levels of satisfaction and/or complaint, facilitating discussion and collaborative decision-making
Evidence passed on from role models and/or experts	Involves facilitating discussion and observation, consultation with experts. Also requires searching the literature for findings from consensus-reaching techniques (focus groups, Delphi surveys, nominal groups techniques and consensus conferences)
Evidence derived from policy documents	Scrutinising documentation, facilitating discussion

Source: From le May (1999).

personal experience and anecdote. Little wonder then that practice requires scrutiny if it is to advance beyond the 'myth, tradition and anecdote' so commonly reported (e.g. Walsh and Ford, 1992; Closs and Cheater, 1994; Maynard, 1994). Thus, despite the emphasis on the importance of research (DoH, 1993a, 1993b; UKCC, 1992b), and the increasing drive towards both research and evidence-based practice (DoH, 1989; National Health Service Executive (NHSE), 1996) it is sad but apparently true that the effectiveness and value of much of nursing practice has never been examined. This being so the increased accountability now expected from nurses demands that clinical practices are carefully evaluated to test their efficacy (Kitson, 1997) and to provide the necessary and credible foundation for professional knowledge and activity (Traynor and Rafferty, 1998). It can, therefore, be claimed that the very future of nursing depends on careful scrutiny of its practices so as to substantiate their use; it is also necessary that inappropriate practices are discarded. It is only when this is achieved that we can claim to have advanced practice to the point where enhanced patient outcome can be ensured and the provision of efficient and economic care can be demonstrated.

Research is, therefore, a professional imperative since, unless nursing actions can be justified, it is likely that the UKCC (1992a) *Code of Professional Conduct*, which states that nurses must ensure that no harm to patients arises from any act or omission on their part, will be breached; without research this cannot be guaranteed (Tordoff, 1998). Similarly, the UKCC (1992b) requires nurses to 'maintain and improve [their] professional competence'; this cannot be achieved without research.

Goals of Nursing Research

Research clearly has the potential to inform nurses not only about nursing but also about physical and scientific issues relevant to nursing practice and so to advance the way that practice is carried out. It may also provide information about relationships and identified interventions and, through these, enable 'beneficial change' to be promoted (DoH, 1989; Bostrum and Suter, 1993; Rizzuto *et al.*, 1994), to 'increase available knowledge by the discovery of new factors or relationships' (Macleod-Clark and Hockey, 1989) or to 'generate and refine clinical nursing interventions' (Rolfe, 1994). Research thus provides the opportunity for nurses to subject their 'art' to scientific scrutiny and to substantiate its claims to provide effective and efficient practice (Thompson, 1998a). It is essential if nursing is to develop a body of knowledge and generate theories to underpin its practice enabling this to be planned and controlled effectively. Achieving this will, as previously shown, enhance professional accountability. Yet, despite the clear need for research, Luker (1997) asserts that nursing has been slow to examine its clinical base and/or develop new or improved interventions.

It can, therefore, be seen that the primary goals of nursing research are to develop the knowledge base underpinning daily practice and to enable practitioners to demonstrate that a specific nursing action or intervention is – on the basis of current best evidence – the most effective means of treating/caring for a patient experiencing a particular clinical problem. At present there is little research to demonstrate the effectiveness of the majority of nursing care activities (World Health Organization, 1994).

However, although nursing research (and research into nursing) requires some disciplinary diversity, there is a tendency for researchers in other disciplines to take over the nursing agenda and make it their own (Mulhall, 1995). Yet, to maintain the focus on nursing, it is essential that nurses themselves participate in research since, although other disciplines may provide some useful evidence, dependence on such work provides only a limited solution to nursing problems as this shifts the emphasis from nursing. Such research may not look at either the problem or the findings in the same way largely due to its different underlying philosophy. Nursing sees patients as more than a 'simple' collection of signs and symptoms, or a particular disease state, and provides care that takes the individual and his needs into account. This holistic perspective necessitates a broader approach that recognises this and considers the synergy that may exist between the individual, his/her disease or illness and the environment. This means that we must often study complex situations and consider multiple variables in seeking to solve clinical problems.

Thus, to advance nursing appropriately we must identify our own areas of concern and design our own research/research strategies to investigate these effectively. In other words, we must undertake careful, systematic enquiries designed to either validate existing knowledge or generate new knowledge about nursing actions and activities. The science of nursing must evolve from, and be responsive to, the needs of nursing practice (Cullum, 1998; Thompson, 1998a). Unless this is the case nursing cannot and will not evolve beyond its current state and practice will remain unchanged.

Paradigms for Nursing Research

As has been shown, nurses in clinical practice must be able to demonstrate a scientific basis for their practice and show that this is grounded by research. The primary aim of such research is, therefore, to determine so-called 'best practice' (Closs and Cheater, 1994) thus enabling nursing to advance. It is, therefore, directed both towards solving problems and generating new knowledge. Hence nursing research studies must be directed towards work investigating the process of delivering care and/or clinical problems encountered during that process (Wilson-Barnett and Robinson, 1989); it should, therefore, generate results that are significant to both nursing practice and patient outcome. Thus research is about the systematic search for understanding and is designed to achieve this objectively in what is described as a 'scientific' (i.e. rigorous) fashion so that its approaches can be seen to be complementary to those of nursing. Like nursing, research is a combination of both art and science in that identifying appropriate questions, which are amenable to research, relies upon both creativity and curiosity (Thompson, 1998a). The way those questions are asked largely determines the method to be used in attempts to answer them.

Science, too, is focused on the search for knowledge and understanding and achieves this in a rational and objective way. Its tenets are, however, often misunderstood in nursing which perceives science as being relevant solely as theory-neutral facts, quantitative approaches and the search for a 'universal truth' (Schumacher and Gortner, 1992; Playle, 1995); it also assumes that such truth exists and can be directly observed. Such research has also been described as reductionist, mechanistic and dehumanising (Thompson, 1998a) and, by reducing facts to numerical data – used to provide information about the 'world', inappropriate to the study of nursing problems. This is as erroneous as the belief that nursing problems can only be studied by means of qualitative approaches more familiar to the social sciences. This dichotomy has lead to marked polarisation in nursing research. As Thompson (1998a) points out, nurses, and nursing researchers, must appreciate that both paradigms have their strengths and their weaknesses; each has its merits and importance in developing nursing practice since neither approach alone is likely to provide an answer to most nursing questions.

Yet one of the problems for nursing lies in the fact that EBP is founded on the belief that the most significant and appropriate evidence is that derived from quantitative research, preferably from the randomised controlled trial (Long and Harrison, 1996). However, although RCTs may constitute the 'ideal' of experimental design they cannot, alone, prove that the right intervention has been provided to the right patient at the right time or even, in the right place (Greenhalgh, 1996). In addition, Schumacher and Gortner (1992) point out that, although this approach to research is used to describe, to test relationships and to examine cause-and-effect relationships, there is no true philosophical or historical basis for believing this is the 'only' (or the 'right') way to do research. Such beliefs are, however, combined with an antagonism, and negative bias, towards qualitative research (Carr, 1994).

It is not, however, surprising that, in nursing, there has been considerable resistance towards the exclusive use of the 'traditional' scientific model of research dependent on either inductive or hypothetico-deductive approaches that are perceived as 'too limiting' to permit full exploration, description or prediction of the nature of nursing (e.g. Rose and Parker, 1994). Thus the natural science paradigm, as a means of studying nursing and nursing problems, is being challenged by those who see nursing only as a human science (e.g. Meleis, 1992) valuing the 'lived experience' and seeking to understand its meaning and values. Therein lies another dilemma for nursing since, if nursing is perceived only as a human science, the questions arising from it must be seen only to reflect its human aspects thus limiting its ability to investigate the wider area of practice and neglecting problems generated by a wide variety of additional factors, theories and interventions. This approach, therefore, overlooks the biological, physiological and medical aspects of care and care delivery; it overlooks the impact of the patient's condition, and/or his 'being' on his response to care and on its outcome.

It seems, therefore, that nursing must embrace a range of research paradigms if practice is to advance since it is quite clear that not all nursing problems can be reduced to a reductionist's scientific approach; it is similarly clear that complex situations cannot be studied only through qualitative research approaches. Since nursing has been defined as the 'diagnosis and treatment of human responses to actual or potential health problems' (American Nurses' Association, 1980, p. 9), and such responses may be physical, biological, emotional or social both research approaches may generate useful knowledge that can be applied to practice. They are complementary one to another and reflect the disciplinary diversity necessary to truly advance the scientific basis of practice. The truth is, of course, that the 'scientific method', reflects all those procedures that scientists currently use or may use in the future (Kaplan, 1964) thus suggesting that there is more than one way to 'do' research' (Munhall, 1983; Thompson, 1998a). Research designs should, therefore, be selected according to their appropriateness and their ability to answer the identified research question and may include either a qualitative or a quantitative approach.

Who Should 'Do' Research?

As we have seen, the aim of research in nursing is to generate knowledge and enhance understanding; it is also directed towards improving the care delivered to patients and the outcome(s) of that care. It is, therefore, clear that all clinical practice should be founded on up-to-date evidence and research findings. This is particularly true if nursing is to meet the demand for demonstrable clinical effectiveness through the provision of evidence-based practice both of which require the integration of expertise and research designed to test specific aspects of practice so as to substantiate their application. There is, therefore, no doubt that the science of nursing must evolve from and be responsive to the needs and demands of nursing practice (Thompson, 1998a) and research priorities should emerge from nurses who are caring for patients (Cullum, 1998) if practice is to advance. Nursing must clearly clarify the nature of its interventions and the outcome(s) of those interventions if it is to demonstrate its contribution to healthcare and to patient outcome(s). The questions then become those of considering who should carry out research into nursing, whether all nurses should 'do' research or whether it is sufficient for the majority to 'simply' understand and implement research findings into their practice.

Research in nursing remains a relatively small enterprise (Mulhall, 1997); the majority of substantive work is located in university departments and specialist research units. Thus, as in many other fields, research is attributed an aura of mystique and authority (Mulhall, 1997) which serves to separate it from the 'real world' of day-to-day practice. Research is seen as an elite activity (Rolfe, 1998) carried out by a highly select group comprising, primarily, academics and emanating from the 'ivory tower' of academia and so perceived to be esoteric and eschewed for its irrelevance to daily work (Luker and Kenrick, 1995; Mulhall, 1997). It is contended that this reflects the 'cultural divide' between researcher and practitioners built on the reductionist approach that separates research from practice attempting to break down the complex whole which is nursing into smaller and seemingly unrelated parts rather than seeing them as component parts of that whole (Mulhall, 1997). This is further exacerbated by the different values and beliefs that exist between education (academic) environments – where the ethos demands research – and the service setting – driven by the need for care delivery. Such disparities clearly perpetuate this division with the unfortunate consequence that research appears to be far removed from the exigencies of daily work in the practice environment. The failure to involve practitioners is reflected in the fact that there is relatively little research that focuses on clinical practice (Burrows and McLeish, 1995). Yet research must be used as a means to benefit practice; it is not an end in itself. It may add to, or modify, experience, common sense or 'traditional' knowledge (Clark, 1988) thus substantiating professional judgement. It is, therefore, relevant to all practitioners who must demonstrate a scientific basis for their practice. This means, in turn, that it is essential that the increased research activity accompanying the move of nurse education into the higher education sector is paralleled by increased awareness and activity at the clinical level (Stevens, 1997) thus helping to place decision-making and professional judgement on a more 'solid footing' (Hicks, 1996).

Yet, although nurses are extensively used as data collectors for research conducted by others, most notably doctors, comparatively small numbers carry out research for themselves (Mulhall, 1997) meaning that there are few role models, and a paucity of expertise, in the clinical environment. Similarly, Hunt (1997) suggests that there is still a somewhat uneasy relationship in many, perhaps the majority of, nurses between their day-to-day activity and research. The focus on evidence-based practice – and therefore research (and utilisation of research) – is now central to healthcare; it is not going to go away! Clinical practitioners should, therefore, grasp the opportunities thus presented to demonstrate the contribution that nursing makes to clinical effectiveness. In other words, to quote McFarlane (1985),

> Research is not a luxury for the academic, but a tool for developing the quality of nursing decisions, prescriptions and actions. Whether as clinicians, educators, managers or researchers, we have a research responsibility; neglect of that responsibility should be classified as professional negligence.

This is not to say that all practitioners should carry out research but that all are required to understand and implement research findings into their practice and that, in this way, research is integral to the credibility of professional practice.

All practitioners must, therefore, be research 'literate', and aware of its importance in promoting change in clinical practice and improvement in patient care. For some practitioners, however, the generation of knowledge should form a central part of their role since this will help to generate pertinent data on which individual care can be based. There can be little argument that research questions arising from practice should be identified by practitioners. The advanced practitioner, however, fulfils a different role a part of which is to promote development(s) by challenging the assumptions underlying current practice and enhancing the scientific basis of that practice; this cannot be achieved unless they become active participants in clinical research. Such practitioners must also disseminate and use research findings to advance practice in their area of expertise, They cannot, however, do this alone and require support both at the organisational level and from others involved in research. It has been argued that such activities are dependent on 'interest, culture and support' (Closs and Cheater, 1994). Thus, both undertaking and utilising research are not only individual issues but require organisational support through, for example, mission statements and policy documents (McGuire, 1990); this must, therefore, occur at all levels of the organisation. Research cannot be viewed as a separate entity that staff perform independently of other duties; the working environment, the care context and its management must, therefore, be considered (Rodgers, 1994). The move towards evidence-based practice, and the demand for clinical effectiveness, are positive moves in this direction.

The support of colleagues who are also involved in research and in changing practice is also important. As a group, active researchers will stimulate creativity and the development of new approaches to solving nursing problems. Sharing problems, debating relevant issues and scrutinising others' work often increases individual productivity and commitment and enables the more experienced to support neophyte researchers. Such an approach enables development of a scientific learning community in which research and development can be discussed and help to enable a theoretical basis for nursing practice to be established; from this practice will advance.

Promoting the Implementation of Research

Evidence-based practice is now central to nursing practice and it is no longer acceptable to base nursing care simply on established practice and tradition (Uitterhoeve and Ambaum, 1999). However, although the transfer of research knowledge into practice is crucial in improving the care delivered to patients the best of way of achieving this is not clear. What is clear is that the availability of research findings is not, in itself, sufficient to guarantee the incorporation into practice (Peckham, 1995; Mulhall, 1997) and the relationship between research findings and their transfer into daily work is clearly complex. It is only too easy for research to become 'uncoupled' from clinical practice (Huth, 1989; Haynes, 1990) as is evidenced by Luker (1992) who asserts that, 'in many instances, there is a gap between what is known and what is practiced'. This, perhaps, reflects, even today, the views of Jacox (1974) who wrote that 'practice is the beginning and end of nursing and anything else which surrounds or cloaks practice is meaningless in comparison'. Thus, seeking out evidence, and evaluating research, may be perceived to detract from practice which is, indeed, the essence of nursing (Berragan, 1998) and reduce the time available for patient care. Yet, without the knowledge derived from research practice cannot advance since developing knowledge in an applied discipline, such as nursing, depends upon extending practical (experiential) knowledge through scientifically based investigations combined with careful observation (Benner, 1984). Benner was, clearly, ahead of her time in integrating the generation of knowledge with experience in advancing patient care and, in this way, was advocating 'evidence-based practice'. The failure to integrate research with practice perhaps reflects the tendency of nurses to adhere to their 'traditional values' – and what they perceive to be important – in the healthcare system rather than using their ability to influence and advance patient care. This contention is supported, in part at least, by the many studies that have explored the reasons why research findings are not used in practice. There is now growing consensus regarding the factors involved many of which have been alluded to throughout this chapter and which can be summarised as shown below:

- The perceived 'cultural divide' between researchers, practitioners and educators (Haines and Jones, 1994; Rolfe, 1998) as well as between practitioners and administrators each of whom has different priorities;

● The belief that research is esoteric and irrelevant to daily practice (Lomas and Haynes, 1988; Luker and Kenrick, 1995; Mulhall, 1997);

● The failure of researchers to 'transform' research findings into innovations specific to a particular patient group or clinical setting (Leske *et al.*, 1994; Mulhall, 1997; le May, 1999);

● Practical/organisational difficulties related to, for example, access to the literature, pressure of work (lack of time) and lack of support (Lomas and Haynes, 1988; Bostrum *et al.*, 1989; Luker and Kenrick, 1995; McIntosh, 1995; le May, 1999).

Similar findings have been obtained in cancer nursing samples. For example, Rutledge *et al.* (1998), using a random sample of 1,100 cancer nurses, rated 28 items in terms of the extent to which they were perceived as barriers to the utilisation of research. Of these, six items were seen to be significant by more than 50 per cent of the sample (see Table 4.5).

The findings shown in Table 4.5 support the many reports of the hindrance to research utilisation arising from a lack of knowledge and understanding of research and the research process as well as difficulty in interpreting the often impenetrable academic style characterising many research papers. Thus researchers often fail to inform practitioners appropriately (Hicks and Hennessy, 1997); this does not, however, negate the

Table 4.5   Top ten barriers to the utilisation of research in oncology nursing practice

Ranking	Barrier	Reporting (%)
1	Unable to understand statistical analysis	62
2	No authority to change patient care	58
3	Lack of time to read research	58
4	No time to implement new ideas	53
5	Implications for practice unclear	53
6	Unable to evaluate the quality of research	47
7	Research not reported clearly	46
8	Relevant literature not in one place	45
9	Lack of support from other staff	45
10	Lack of co-operation from physicians	43

Source: From Rutledge *et al.* (1998).

fact that there is a lack of high-quality published research that has the ability to alter/change practice (Smith, 1996).

At the same time, however, the lack of confidence in nurses to both conduct and evaluate research also significantly impacts on the ability to implement research findings. This, in all probability, reflects the lack of an academic (and, therefore, research) tradition within nursing which is now playing 'catch up' with other disciplines. To do this successfully requires significant cultural change to overcome the entrenched attitudes resulting in reluctance to embrace any activities that are not firmly embedded in direct caring activity and patient care (Hicks, 1995); such attitudes are peculiarly resistant to change (McIntosh, 1995).

It is, therefore, clear that strategies are needed to promote both dissemination and implementation of research and research findings. To date, nursing has largely relied upon a 'passive unplanned diffusion process' rather than a 'planned and systematic process' (Crosswaite and Curtice, 1994). The former is somewhat haphazard depending on the ability, skill and interest of individuals or small groups of practitioners; it also lacks a clear target and works well only when those involved are highly motivated. To rely on such a process is unlikely to ensure that practice will move forward or to enhance care delivery. That said, however, implementation cannot occur unless defined processes of dissemination are in place. This first necessitates consideration of the availability of relevant information. There has, undoubtedly, been a significant increase in the number of journals including nursing research over the past twenty years thus increasing the availability of a significant amount of relevant information. Indeed, the literature is now so vast that 'information overload' is a significant problem (Deykin and Haines, 1996). There is no doubt that the increasing number of journals means that the number of clinically important studies are spread thinly across a vast number of journals; it is not, therefore, surprising if practitioners are overwhelmed (Haynes and Haines, 1998). This vast literature has, in turn, increased the availability of equivocal findings and enhances the difficulty of implementation. Many healthcare professionals have neither the time nor the resources to keep up with the amount of literature available; many also lack the ability to evaluate it and take from it what is relevant or meaningful to their practice. It is for this reason that comprehensive and unbiased summaries of research findings (systematic reviews) (Mulrow, 1994) are invaluable in helping to increase nurses' confidence in the findings of research and also the ability and willingness to implement them (Dickson and Cullum, 1996). Journals focusing on the use of evidence to guide practice are also increasingly available (Dickson and Entwhistle, 1996) making access to relevant information easier.

This has been supported through several national initiatives such as the Cochrane Collaboration on Effective Professional Practice and the NHS

Centre for Reviews and Dissemination, both of which act to produce and maintain systematic reviews and maintain a core database of up-to-date evidence of the effects of healthcare. These are robust resources for all healthcare practitioners providing highly controlled and rigorous reviews of the evidence and offering a good 'short cut' for nurses wishing to develop their practice through research. Nursing libraries will have abstracts of such work, and may provide access through CD-roms, together with that of the Database of Abstracts of Reviews of Effectiveness (DARE). However, the vast majority of topics reviewed to date centre on clinical treatments for different pathologies which is, perhaps, not surprising since most systematic reviews deal exclusively with RCTs. Some reviews included in the Cochrane Collaboration do, however, have a broader remit and some specifically address nursing practice.

Such approaches, while clearly increasing the amount of information in both the public and the professional domains do not, of necessity, bring this to the attention of individual practitioners so that strategies directed at the individual and the local level are also needed. There is considerable evidence to suggest that practitioners do not know about research findings (e.g. Dickson, 1996) yet a variety of mechanisms exist for making research available, including increasing access to journals and libraries and enhanced access to computer searching (e.g. Champion and Leach, 1989; Bostrum and Wilse, 1994) and the introduction of clinical liaison nurses who act as intermediaries in the accessing of research findings relevant to practice in specific areas (Akinsanya, 1994; Lacey, 1994); such activity can be enhanced by the role of the advanced practitioner.

However, having accessed information it is up to individual practitioners to evaluate research to determine its validity and its generalisability to their practice setting. It is essential that the relevance of research findings to individual settings is demonstrated and that research is validated in the context of that setting. In this way evidence derived from research is used to augment the tacit knowledge of practitioners (i.e. evidence that is not in the scientific literature but that is well known to practitioners (Carroll, 1988). To make this possible requires that researchers make their findings available and accessible to practitioners. Academic researchers are, undoubtedly, in a difficult position since, to maintain their credibility in academia and the funding for their institutions, they are required to publish their work in peer-reviewed journals; this, in turn, determines not only the nature of the research they undertake but also the 'language' they use to report it (Crosswaite and Curtice, 1994). This creates still further problems for practitioners since research reported for academic scrutiny tends to be reported in research journals while clinicians tend to read other (professional) journals. Moreover, practitioners may find it difficult to understand the implications of particular research studies for their practice. Thus, to make their work relevant to practitioners academics must consider how to overcome such problems by making their research accessible and highlighting its clinical relevance. They must develop dissemination strategies that meet the needs of both academia and practice; this then is the challenge to academics.

A second challenge focuses on the involvement of practitioners in research. If, as has been suggested, research questions should arise from practice (Cullum, 1998; Thompson, 1998a) it is clearly necessary that academics and practitioners work together to promote research and disseminate its findings. Opportunities for such developments must be actively sought if evidence is to be used in practice and ensure progress towards demonstrable clinical effectiveness.

Where Do We Go From Here?

The preceding discussion has clearly revealed that remarkably little current nursing practice is based on research findings and, even within cancer nursing, many practices continue to be based on intuition, tradition and/or untested theory (Robinson, 1999). Little wonder then that the need for strategies to promote research has been emphasised (Corner, 1993; RCN, 1996) or that it is recommended that nursing research becomes an integral part of the overall programme of R&D within cancer centres (RCN, 1996). This may, however, be easier said than done in the light of the existence of the many barriers to research and research utilisation. Advanced practitioners, and other nursing leaders, are in a position to both facilitate and promote research and the utilisation of its findings. Since the barriers are well known, many can be anticipated so that mechanisms can be established to overcome them and minimise their impact in individual practice settings.

Nurse managers are in key positions and so able to facilitate or to hinder research activity (Cullum, 1996) and should promote collaboration between those undertaking research and those delivering patient care. Such collaboration will help to ensure that researchers answer questions relevant to practitioners and encourage practitioners to implement research findings. Managers must promote the dissemination and implementation of research findings if they are to facilitate evidence-based practice and demonstrable clinical effectiveness and so meet the demands of clinical governance. They must create time within the practice environment to enable practitioners to access and read research. Advances in technology can provide quick and often inexpensive access to high quality research evidence (Hersh, 1996; Sackett *et al.*, 1997); such technology must be available to practitioners so that the practice of evidence-based nursing becomes increasingly feasible.

Policy-makers, particularly when involved in nursing, must ensure that they base such policy on clearly established – and rigorously evaluated – evidence (Cullum, 1996). For too long, policy has been driven by a range of non-evidence-based factors including historical, cultural and ideological influences (Hunter and Polit, 1992; Haynes and Haines, 1998); this must be overcome. Thus policy-makers also need access to the best available evidence as well as the ability to evaluate its relevance for their policy areas. Research should drive policy just as it should drive practice.

Researchers must conduct research in collaboration not only with practitioners – although this is central to practice development – but also, where appropriate or necessary, with other disciplines and professions to produce research which is relevant to practice but also of high quality and demonstrable scientific rigour. Such an approach will support the development of clinically effective and integrated patient care. Finally, researchers must, as previously described, make their findings both available and accessible to practitioners; they must report their work in journals appropriate to practitioners, in simple and straightforward language and in ways that clearly identify the implications of their findings to practice.

To achieve such changes necessitates, in turn, considerable changes in the culture of not only nursing itself but also within academia and the health services as a whole. A systematic process, designed to facilitate both evidence-based practice and clinical effectiveness is crucial so that strategies for change must be developed at all levels of healthcare if practice development is to take place. To be effective, such strategies must clearly involve approaches designed to enhance research awareness among not only clinicians but all those involved in healthcare and increase the dissemination of appropriate and relevant research findings. It is only in this way that practice can advance through research.

References

Akinsanya, J. (1994) Making research useful to the practice nurse. *Journal of Advanced Nursing*, 19, 174–9.

American Nursing Association (1980) *Nursing: A Social Policy Statement*. Kansas City, MO: ANA.

Appleby, J., K. Walshe and C. Ham (1995) *Acting on the Evidence*. Research Paper 17. Birmingham: National Association of Health Authorities and Trusts.

Benner, P. (1984) *From Novice to Expert: Excellence and Power in Clinical Nursing Practice*. Menlo Park, CA: Addison-Wesley.

Berragan, L. (1998) Nursing practice draws upon several different ways of knowing. *Journal of Clinical Nursing*, 7, 209–17.

Blumenthal, D. (1994) The variation phenomenon in 1994. *New England Journal of Medicine*, 531, 1017–18.

) Issues in measuring outcomes of controlled trials in nursing: a *Health Care*, 6, 2–6.

Dougall and D. Hargis (1989) Staff nurses' attitudes towards survey. *Journal of Advanced Nursing*, 14, 915–22.

3) Research utilization: making the link to practice. *Journal of* 34.

ing the gap between research and practice. *Journal of Nursing*

5) A model for research-based practice. *Journal of Clinical*

ness of qualitative and quantitative research: what method ing, 20, 716–21.

ledge in problem solving in the clinical setting. *Nurse*

es related to research utilisation in nursing: an empir- rsing, 14, 705–10.

ctive practice: reviewing the issues and refocusing the dies, 33(2), 171–80.

e. *Professional Nurse*, 3, 344–7.

a retrograde step? The importance of pluralism in alth care. *Journal of Clinical Nursing*, 6, 175–8.

n of nursing research: culture, interest and support.

nursing research in cancer care. *European Journal of*

ing research results – the challenge of bridging the h *Promotion International*, 9, 289–96.

Management, 3(4), 14–16.

sing Management, 5(3), 32–5.

in England. London: DoH.

A Research and Development Strategy for the NHS.

Department of Health (1993a) *Report of the Taskforce on the Strategy for Research in Nursing, Midwifery and Health Visiting*. London: DoH.

Department of Health (1993b) *Research for Health*. London: DoH.

Department of Health (2001) *Strategy for Nursing Research*. London: DoH.

Department of Health and Social Security (1972) *Report of the Committee on Nursing (Cmd 5115, Briggs Report)* London: DHSS.

Deykin, D. and A. Haines (1996) Promoting the use of research findings, in M. Peckham and R. Smith (eds), *The Scientific Basis of Health Services*. London: BMJ Publishing.

DiCenso, A., N. Cullum and D. Ciliska (1998) Implementing evidence-based nursing: some misconceptions. *Evidence-Based Nursing*, 1(20), 38–40.

Dickson, R. (1996) Dissemination and implementation: the wider picture. *Nurse Researcher*, 4(1), 5–14.

Dickson, R. and N. Cullum (1996) Systematic reviews: how to use the information. *Nursing Standard*, 10(2), 32.

Dickson, R. and V. Entwhistle (1996) Systematic reviews: keeping up with research evidence. *Nursing Standard*, 10(14), 32.

Foundation of Nursing Studies (1996) *Reflection for Action*. London: Foundation of Nursing Studies.

French, P. (1999) The development of evidence-based nursing. *Journal of Advanced Nursing*, 29(1), 72–8.

Gould, D. (1999) Evidence-based care: issues in biomedical nursing. *Journal of Clinical Nursing*, 8, 121–2.

Gray, J.A.M. (1997) *Evidence-Based Healthcare*. Edinburgh: Faber & Faber.

Greenhalgh, T. (1996) Is my practice evidence-based?: should be answered in qualitative, as well as quantitative terms. *British Medical Journal*, 313, 957–8.

Haynes, B. and A. Haines (1998) Getting research findings into practice: barriers and bridges to evidence-based clinical practice. *British Medical Journal*, 317, 273–6.

Haines, A. and R. Jones (1994) Implementing findings of research. *British Medical Journal*, 308, 1488–92.

Hardey, M. and A. Mulhall (1994) *Nursing Research, Theory and Practice*. London: Chapman & Hall.

Haynes, R.B. (1990) Loose connections between peer-reviewed clinical journals. *Annals of Internal Medicine*, 113, 724–8.

Hersh, W. (1996) Evidence-based medicine and the internet. *ACP Journal Club*, 125, A14–16.

Hicks, C.(1995) The shortfall in published research: a study of nurses' research and publication activities. *Journal of Advanced Nursing*, 21(3), 594–604.

Hicks, C. (1996) Nurse researcher: a study of a contradiction in terms? *Journal of Advanced Nursing*, 24(2), 357–63.

Hicks, C. and D. Hennessy (1997) Mixed messages in nursing research: their contribution to the persisting hiatus between evidence and practice. *Journal of Advanced Nursing*, 25, 595–601.

Holmes, S. (1991) Clinical leadership: a role for the advanced practitioner? *Journal of Advances in Health and Nursing Care*, 1, 3–20.

Hunt, J. (1997) Towards evidence-based practice. *Nursing Management*, 4(2), 14–17.

Hunter, D.J. and C. Polit (1992) Development of health services research: perspectives from Britain and the United States. *Journal of Public Health Medicine*, 14, 163–8.

Huth, E. (1989) The underused medical literature. *Annals of Internal Medicine*, 110, 99–100.

Jacox, A. (1974) Theory construction in nursing: an overview. *Nursing Research*, 23(1), 4–13.

Kaplan, A. (1964) *The Conduct of Inquiry: Methodology for Behavioural Science*. New York: Chandler.

Kitson, A. (1997) Lessons from the 1996 research assessment exercise. *Nurse Researcher*, 4, 81–93.

Lacey, G.A. (1994) Research utilization in practice – a pilot study. *Journal of Advanced Nursing*, 19, 987–95.

le May, A. (1999) *Evidence-based practice*, Nursing Times Clinical Monographs No. 2. London: Nursing Times Books.

le May, A., C. Alexander and A. Mulhall (1998) Research-based practice: practitioners' and managers' view. *Managing Clinical Nursing*, 2(3), 87–92.

Leske, J.S., K. Whiteman, T.A. Freichels and J.M. Pearcy (1994) Using clinical innovations for research-based care. *Clinical Issues in Critical Care Nursing*, 5, 103–14.

Lomas, J. and R.B. Haynes (1988) A taxonomy and critical review of tested strategies for the application of clinical practice recommendations: from 'official' to 'individual'. *American Journal of Preventative Medicine*, 4 (Suppl), 77–95.

Long, A. (1996) Health services research – a radical approach to cross the research and development divide, in M. Baker and S. Kirk (eds) *Research and Development for the NHS: Evidence, Evaluation and Effectiveness*. Oxford: Radcliffe Medical Press.

Long, A. and S. Harrison (1996) *The balance of evidence. Evidence-based Decision Making*. London: Macmillan Magazines.

Lorentzon, M. (1995) Multidisciplinary collaboration: lifeline or drowning pool for nurse researchers? (Guest Editorial). *Journal of Advanced Nursing*, 22, 825.

Luker, K. (1992) Research and development in nursing. *Journal of Advanced Nursing*, 17, 1151–2.

Luker, K. (1997) Research and the configuration of nursing services. *Journal of Clinical Nursing*, 6, 259–67.

Luker, K. and M. Kenrick (1995) Towards knowledge-based practice; an evaluation of a method of dissemination. *International Journal of Nursing Studies*, 32(1), 59–67.

Maynard, A. (1994) Knowledge based – not blindly based. *Nursing Management*, 1(4), 9.

McFarlane, J. (1980) *Accountability*. Report of the Royal College of Nursing. London: RCN.

McFarlane, J. (1985) Contemporary challenges in education for the caring professions: education for nursing, midwifery, and health visiting. *British Medical Journal*, 291(6490), 268–71.

McGuire, J.M. (1990) Putting nursing research findings into practice: research utilisation as an aspect of management. *Journal of Advanced Nursing*, 15, 614–20.

McIntosh, J. (1995) Barriers to research implementation. *Nurse Researcher*, 2, 83–91.

McLeod Clark, J. and L. Hockey (1989) *Further Research for Nursing*. London: Scutari Press.

McSherry, R. (1997) What do registered nurses and midwives fear and know about research? *Journal of Advanced Nursing*, 25, 985–9.

Meleis, A. (1992) Directions for nursing theory development in the 21st century. *Nursing Science Quarterly*, 5, 3.

Mulhall, A. (1995) Nursing research: what difference does it make? *Journal of Advanced Nursing*, 21, 576–83.

Mulhall, A. (1997) Nursing research: our world not theirs? *Journal of Advanced Nursing*, 25, 969–76.

Mulrow, C. (1994) Rationale for systematic reviews. *British Medical Journal*, 309, 597–9.

Munhall, P. (1983) Methodological fallacies: a critical self-appraisal. *Advances in Nursing Science*, 5(4), 41–9.

Naylor, C.D. (1995) Grey zones of clinical practice: some limits to evidence-based medicine. *Lancet*, 345, 840–2.

NHS Executive (1996) *Promoting Clinical Effectiveness: a framework for action and through the NHS.* London: DoH.

Peckham, M. (1991) Research and development for the National Health Service. *Lancet*, 338, 367–71.

Peckham, M. (1995) The new role of R&D: the challenge for NHS Boards. *Health Director*, 24, 8–9.

Playle, J. (1995) Humanism and positivism in nursing: contradiction and conflicts. *Journal of Advanced Nursing*, 22, 979–84.

Rizzuto, C., J. Bostrum, W.N. Suter, and W.C. Chenitz (1994) Predictors of nurses involvement in research activities. *Western Journal of Nursing Research*, 16, 193–204.

Robinson, L. (1999) Research for cancer nursing (Editorial). *European Journal of Cancer Nursing*, 3, 119–20.

Rodgers, C. (1994) An explanatory study of research utilisation by nurses in general medical and surgical wards. *Journal of Advanced Nursing*, 20, 904–11.

Rolfe, G. (1994) Towards a new model of nursing research. *Journal of Advanced Nursing*, 19, 969–75.

Rolfe, G. (1998) The theory-practice gap in nursing: from research-based practice to practitioner-based research. *Journal of Advanced Nursing*, 28, 672–9.

Rose, F. and D. Parker (1994) Nursing: an integration of art and science within the experiences of the practitioner. *Journal of Advanced Nursing*, 20, 1004–10.

Rosenberg, X. and A. Donald (1995) Evidence-based medicine: an approach to clinical problem solving. *British Medical Journal*, 310, 1122–3.

Royal College of Nursing (1996) *A Structure for Cancer Nursing Services.* London: RCN.

Rutledge, D.N., M. Ropka, P.E. Greene, L. Nail and K.N. Mooney (1998) Barriers to research utilization for oncology staff nurses and nurse managers/clinical nurse specialists. *Oncology Nursing Forum*, 23, 497–506.

Sackett, D.L., W.M. Rosenberg, J.A.M. Gray, R.B. Haynes and W.S. Richardson (1996) Evidence-based medicine: what it is and what it is not. *British Medical Journal*, 312, 71–2.

Sackett, D.L., S.R. Richardson, S. Rosenberg and R.B. Haynes (1997) *Evidence-based medicine: how to practice and to teach EBM.* London: Churchill Livingstone.

Schober, J.E. (1995) Nursing: Current issues and the patients' perspective, in J.E. Schober and S.M. Hinchliffe (eds), *Towards Advanced Nursing Practice: Key Concepts for Health Care.* London: Arnold.

Schumacher, K. and S. Gortner (1992) (Mis)conceptions and reconceptions about traditional sciences. *Advances in Nursing Science*, 14(4), 1–11.

Smith, R. (1996) Editor's choice: more better research now. *British Medical Journal*, 313, 1201.

Spitzer, A. (1998) Nursing in the health care system of the postmodern world: crossroads, paradoxes and complexity. *Journal of Advanced Nursing*, 28, 164–71.

Stevens, J. (1997) Improving integration between research and practice as a means of developing evidence-based health care. *NT Research*, 2, 7–15.

Thompson, D. (1998a) The art and science of research in clinical nursing, in B. Roe and C. Webb (eds), *Research and Development in Clinical Nursing Practice.* London: Whurr.

Thompson, D. (1998b) Why evidence-based nursing? *Nursing Standard*, 13(9), 58–9.

Tordoff, C. (1998) From research to practice: a review of the literature. *Nursing Standard*, 12(25), 34–7.

Traynor, M. and A.M. Rafferty (1997) *The NHS R & D Context for Nursing Research: a Working Paper.* London: Centre for Policy in Nursing Research.

Traynor, M. and A.M. Rafferty (1998) *Nursing Research and the Higher Education Context.* London: Centre for Policy in Nursing Research.

Uitterhoeve, R. and B. Ambaum (1999) Surviving the era of evidence-based nursing practice: implementation of a research utilization model in practice. *European Journal of Cancer Nursing*, 3, 185–91.

United Kingdom Central Council for Nursing, Midwifery and Health Visiting (1992a) *The Code of Professional Conduct*, 3rd edn. London: UKCC.

United Kingdom Central Council for Nursing, Midwifery and Health Visiting (1992b) *The Future of Professional Practice – the Council's Standards for Education and practice following Registration*. London: UKCC.

Walsh, M. and P. Ford (1992) *Nursing Rituals* (Second edition). Oxford: Butterworth-Heinemann.

Watson, J. (1998) Foreword in R. McMahon and A. Pearson (eds), *Nursing as Therapy*, 2nd edn. Cheltenham: Stanley Thornes.

White, S.J. (1997) Evidence-based practice and nursing: the new panacea? *British Journal of Nursing*, 6, 175–8.

Wilson-Barnett, J. and J. Robinson (eds) (1989) Directions in Nursing Research: ten years of progress at London University. London: Scutari.

World Health Organization (1994) *Nursing Beyond the year 2000*: Report of a WHO Study Group. Technical Report Series 842. Geneva: WHO.

Part II

This part starts with a synthesis of the evidence relating to current innovations in cancer treatment. Chapter 5, indicates that the next ten years will be a period of very rapid change in cancer care. The issues arising from this technological expansion are identified as they impact upon patients, service delivery and professional nursing care.

The main focus of Chapter 6 is family support. Through an appreciation of the evidence of the needs and problems of families, it is apparent that there remains a lot to be achieved with regard to family care when one person has cancer. The authors explore here the concept of 'expanded nursing practice', as a means of improving family outcomes. Family Nursing 'blurs the boundaries' between 'nursing' and 'therapy' and its usefulness for cancer and palliative care is critically explored.

Chapters 7, 8 and 9 address some of the most fundamentally difficult issues in cancer and palliative care. In Chapter 7 the authors explore the concept of spiritual distress, describing the search for meaning which often accompanies a diagnosis of cancer. The nurse's engagement with others in spiritual distress is seen as complex and advanced work and the authors attempt to describe the essence of a caring, response without resorting to an idyllic and utopian view of the nurse–patient relationship.

In Chapter 8, Nurse and Chaplain respectively, examine advancing practice in palliative and cancer care in relation to ethics. The factors which affect and effect the 'quality' of ethical decision-making are thoughtfully explored as they have direct relevance to skilled nursing. This theme is continued in Chapter 9 which focuses very specifically upon notions of suffering and dying well. This is a clear, informed analysis of end of life decisions which examines the 'fraught' ethical dilemmas involved in the notion of a good death.

5

Innovations in Cancer Therapeutics

CATHERINE M. JACK

Introduction

In the past thirty years there have been relatively modest improvements in overall survival for the majority of cancer patients with the common types of epithelial malignancy. Patients with some of the rarer types of malignant disease – childhood lymphoblastic leukaemia, Hodgkin's lymphoma and germ cell tumours – now have a greatly improved prognosis. Progress in these areas has largely been the result of slow and painstaking accumulation of data through successive clinical trials rather than from the dramatic discovery of new drugs or other treatments. Indeed, during this period there have been relatively few new cytotoxic drugs. Progress has also been made in defining the role of various surgical proced-ures. Many patients with breast cancer now have conservative surgery rather than more radical procedures without prejudice to their outcome (Park et al., 2000; Ogawa et al., 2000).

There have also been important developments in the supportive care of cancer patients and there is much greater awareness of quality of life issues and the importance of palliation and disease control in those who will not be cured of their disease. Improvements in nursing care have focused on assessment, symptom management and the psychological support of the patient throughout their illness. There is now much greater openness in communication between patients and their carers. This has been accom-panied by widespread discussion of cancer related issues in the media.

Standards of practice that incorporate these many incremental improve-ments in care can lead to considerably better outcomes and quality of life for patients. This is clearly shown in comparison between cancer centres and between countries. In general, outcomes within the United Kingdom are poor in comparison with other European countries and with North America (Berrino *et al.*, 1998). If the results of the best centres in practice were achieved across the United Kingdom, this alone would significantly improve outcomes in morbidity and mortality.

Probably the most significant development in cancer research in the past twenty years has been the growth in the understanding of the cellular and molecular biology of the cancer cell. Major progress has been achieved and this continues at an accelerating pace. The goal is to be able to describe the clinical behaviour of individual tumours in terms of acquired genetic abnormalities in the cancer cell. It is this knowledge coupled with the growth of novel techniques in biotechnology, that is now beginning to have a major impact on patient care and in the coming years will transform the practice of oncology.

The purpose of this chapter is to provide a brief outline of some of these developments and to highlight the new challenges that nurses working in cancer care will face in the years ahead.

Understanding the Nature of the Cancer Cell

Until the mid-1980s cancer was often defined as an uncontrolled growth of cells. Not only is this incorrect, but such definitions contained little useful information since almost nothing was known about the control of normal cell growth. It was suspected that genetic damage was a key factor in causing the development of cancer but little was known about the precise mechanisms that resulted in the acquisition of malignant characteristics by a particular cell.

The ability to maintain cells in culture and the experimental work that followed was to dramatically change this situation. A key insight came from the study of ribonucleic acid (RNA) tumour viruses. Animal viruses that could cause malignant disease were described by Peyton Rous in 1912 and were then largely forgotten for several decades. After infecting a cell, the RNA virus makes a deoxyribonucleic acid (DNA) copy of its RNA genome, which is then able to insert itself into one of the host chromosomes. A simple but crucial observation was that when RNA tumour viruses were added to cells in culture, some strains of virus appeared to be much more efficient than others at causing transformation of the target cells. Transformation of cultured cells is a similar process to the production of tumours in whole animals. Investigation of this phenomenon revealed that the efficient viruses carried an extra gene that, by itself, could transform cells. The other viruses only transformed cells if they inserted themselves into certain critical locations on host chromosomes. This by itself would have been a major discovery but it soon become apparent that the transforming genes found in viruses were near replicas of normal genes present in all cells. These genes had been accidentally copied during virus replication in an infected cell and become part of the viral genome. Viruses that did not carry these genes were able to transform cells if they became inserted close to one of these genes and altered its expression (Butel, 2000). This was a crucial observation in helping to identify normal cellular genes which underlie normal processes in cell division and differentiation and can become abnormally expressed in cancer cells.

Ribonucleic acid tumour viruses are not common causes of cancer in humans or in wild animal populations. Examples include a type of T-cell leukaemia found in Japan and the Caribbean caused by HTLV 1 (Manns *et al.*, 1999; Greaves *et al.*, 1984) and the feline leukaemia virus which is common in domestic cats in the United Kingdom. However, these studies led to the model that now underpins a large part of contemporary cancer research. The key elements of this model are:

(1) Cancer is caused by acquired genetic change.

(2) These changes cause altered expression in a critical set of genes that change the behaviour of the cell.

(3) Usually several different genes need to be affected before a clinically apparent tumour develops.

Subsequent studies have characterised the nature and function of many of the critical genes that are disregulated in cancer cells. The proteins coded by these genes are often involved in signalling pathways that transmit information from the cell environment to the nucleus causing changes in the pattern of gene expression (Kinoshita, 1990; Madhukar and Trosko, 1997; Weinberg, 1983; Bishop, 1982). The effect of these stimuli include triggering a cell to divide, to change its function or in some cases to die. The cell receives signals from its environment through cell surface receptors that are able to bind specific hormones or cytokines (short-range messenger molecules secreted by other cells in the vicinity). When a receptor molecule binds its specific cytokine, it is able to activate other signalling molecules within the cell. The effects of many different receptor pathways are integrated by cross inhibition or augmentation with the end effect being a change in the activity of a nuclear transcription factor. These are molecules that bind to specific sites on DNA and result in changes in gene expression. In the cancer cell genetic changes may alter the activity of components of this pathway. Receptors may be active in the absence of cytokines or transcription factor may be present in abnormally large amounts and be partially free from external regulation. An example of this type of abnormality, found in many types of cancer cell, is mutation of the *ras* proteins

(Pincus *et al.*, 2000). These proteins act as a switch linking cell surface receptors to the signalling pathway. Mutation leads to the switch being effectively locked in the on position, leading to false signals being transmitted to the cell nucleus.

A second crucial pathway that is affected in cancer is the cell cycle. This is the process that regulates DNA replication and cell division (Wagner, 1998; Lundberg and Weinberg, 1999; Weinberg, 1996). To complete a cycle of division the cell must pass through a checkpoint before the replication of DNA can begin. This requires both signals from the external environment and absence of damage to DNA. Cells with damaged DNA are inhibited from proceeding to DNA replication until the damage is repaired. If this does not occur the cell's death programme is triggered. A key molecule in this pathway is *p53*. Mutation or deletion of this molecule is one of the commonest genetic abnormalities found in human cancers (Tarapore and Fukasawa, 2000; Tokino and Nakamura, 2000). When *p53* is defective, the cell is able to proceed to division with damaged DNA which accelerates the process of further genetic change (Chen *et al.*, 1999; Komiya *et al.*, 1999).

An important idea in cellular biology is the recognition that cell death is an active process that involves activation of a range of enzymes that degrade the cell and result in its safe disposal. Cell death is a key element in normal development and for the removal of senescent or abnormal cells (Lundberg and Weinberg, 1999). Most anti-cancer drugs and radiotherapy act by activating programmed cell death (Denmeade and Isaacs, 1996; Ross, 1999). The cell death pathway is also affected by a range of genetic abnormalities seen in cancer cells. Normal lymphocytes die unless they receive survival signals from their environment. These signals induce the expression of *bcl-2*, which is a potent inhibitor of cell death. In some B-cell lymphomas, a chromosomal translocation results in the *bcl-2* gene moving from chromosome 18 to the immunoglobulin gene locus on chromosome 14. The expression of *bcl-2* is now under control of the factors that regulate the immunoglobulin gene rather than the bcl-2 gene itself and cells continue to express *bcl-2* protein and survive, even when survival signals are absent. Affected cells live much longer than their normal counterparts and are able to accumulate further genetic defects leading to the development of lymphoma (Meijerink, 1997; Vaandrager *et al.*, 2000).

The Development of Techniques in Biotechnology

The ability to isolate and manipulate DNA is one of the major achievements of the twentieth century and will be a key element in the development of new diagnostic and therapeutic techniques in the twenty-first century.

DNA consists of long strands of four bases – A, T, C and G – joined together by a backbone of sugar and phosphate links. The order of the bases is the 'genetic code' that cells are able to translate into the synthesis of specific protein molecules. DNA usually exists in a double stranded form with two complementary strands in which A is paired with T and C with G. One of the key discoveries in biotechnology was the recognition of a group of bacterial enzymes that cut DNA only at specific sequences of bases. These sequences are relatively rare and so digesting extracted cellular DNA with one of these enzymes produces large fragments of predictable size. Some of these enzymes do not cut each strand at the same point, producing 'sticky ends' that will tend to join with other fragments cut by the same enzyme.

This observation has major implications because it allows DNA extracted from different types of cell, which has been digested using the same enzyme, to be readily joined together. This is the basis of genetic cloning in which fragments of human cellular DNA can be joined to bacterial DNA. This is then re-inserted into bacteria that can be grown in culture to form a large mass of organisms, all containing the same fragment of human DNA. Bacteria can be readily induced to express human genes transfected in this way, producing very large amounts of human protein that can be harvested and purified. Drugs commonly used in oncology such as G-CSF and alpha interferon are now routinely produced in this way. Cloned DNA is frequently used as molecular probes to analyse cancer cells for specific genetic abnormalities.

A major development of this technology was the invention of the *polymerase chain reaction* (PCR) (Mullis, 1990). This is a technique that allows specific segments of whole cellular DNA to be replicated to produce a quantity sufficient for analysis or further cloning. It is now relatively simple to determine the sequence of a segment of DNA that has been produced in a PCR reaction and to detect the presence of mutations or other abnormalities.

The second major technology used in cancer diagnosis and treatment is the production of *monoclonal antibodies* (Erickson, 1990; Milstein, 1980). Antibodies recognise specific shapes on the surface of protein and other molecules. These shapes are determined by the amino acid sequence and some will be unique to that protein. It is therefore possible to produce antibodies that will bind with very high specificity to a particular protein or other molecules. Individual B-lymphocytes are capable of producing only a single type of antibody. Animals injected with a purified protein produce antibodies against various parts of the molecule with varying specificity and affinity of binding. After a period, the immune response subsides and level of the antibody of interest in the animal's serum decreases. The technique of monoclonal antibody production overcomes many of these problems. A mouse is immunised with the protein of interest and after the immune response develops, the animal's spleen is removed and disaggregated to produce a suspension of B-lymphocytes producing antibodies to the injected protein. These cells are then mixed with a cell line derived from a mouse myeloma that can be maintained in permanent cell culture. The splenic lymphocytes are then fused with the myeloma cell to produce hybrid cells. These continue to produce the antibody that was being produced by the B-lymphocyte, but also have the property of perpetual growth in culture acquired from the myeloma cell. These hybrid cells are diluted to the extent that an individual culture will contain only a single cell. These cells divide repeatedly to produce a clone of cells capable of secreting a unique antibody. Clones producing antibodies that are of interest can be then selected and established in culture to produce unlimited amounts of antibody. Monoclonal antibodies produced in this way are essential for the accurate diagnosis of cancer and a number are now being used directly in the treatment of patients, for example *Anti – CD20* used in the treatment of lymphoma (Maloney *et al.*, 1997; Jurcic *et al.*, 1997; Link and Weiner, 1998).

One of the most complicated and difficult practical problems in biotechnology concerns the application of patent law. Until recently, patents have been associated with inventions and tangible products such as new drugs or pieces of equipment. However, the biotechnology industry is pushing back these frontiers, with attempts to patent human genes, types of cell and even possibly whole animals. Where these applications are successful, the use of information such as a genetic sequence in diagnosis or treatment of patients will attract a royalty payment. Many individuals find the idea of patenting a human cell or gene objectionable. However, the contrary argument is that without a financial return on the intellectual capital expended, the pace of development in this area will be impeded. There is little doubt that effective novel therapies and diagnostics will command a premium price that will be set by the global market for these products. This may lead to considerable cost pressures on healthcare budgets and potentially very difficult choices on which patients to treat. Such pressures are already apparent in several areas of oncology.

Genetic manipulation of plants or animals, especially humans, is seen by many as dangerous or even immoral and the biotechnology industry may be the subject of mistrust and suspicion. Some patients may be reluctant to accept therapies based on these techniques. However, many other patients may have concerns about safety or other aspects of the treatment. It is in this situation that it is critical that the patient has access to balanced and authoritative information that will facilitate informed choices.

The Changing Approach to Cancer Diagnosis

At present the diagnosis of cancer is based on histopathological criteria, which are the recognition of microscopic changes in the appearance of cells and in the structure of tissues. Classifications and systems of grading of tumours have been developed that give some information on prognosis and tumour spread. Such classifications are listed in the *International Classification of Diseases for Oncology* and in many other publications. Most of these criteria have developed empirically over the past century and many predate the current era in the understanding the nature of the cancer cell.

In the next decade there is likely to be profound change in this area. It is now possible to produce an array of DNA probes on a 'chip' of glass 1cm^2 that allows samples of cells to be characterised in terms of the expression of up 10,000 different genes. The processing of these 'chips' is fast and automated. This technology will allow some cancers to be accurately diagnosed on minimal samples taken with the aid of a sophisticated imaging device or possibly even on a peripheral blood sample (Wallace, 1997; Kurian *et al.*, 1999; Henn, 1999).

These developments will extend much further than simply replacing microscopy with automated molecular methods. As knowledge advances, an individual disease will be classified not on the basis of empirical criteria but on the fundamental genetic abnormalities that are causing the aberrant behaviour of the tumour cells. This will include abnormalities of cell proliferation, cell signalling and cell death pathways as well as factors such as secretion of enzymes and cell adhesion that determine metastatic potential. These developments are essential to the development of tumour specific therapies. A practical problem, that is already apparent in some areas, is that different diagnostic standards may apply in different centres depending on access to advanced diagnostic facilities. This not only affects the standard of care, but also can make comparison of results difficult.

The Changing Approach to Cancer Screening

Developments in biotechnology will have a major impact on the process of cancer screening. At present, breast and cervical screening are the only national cancer screening programmes in the United Kingdom. Screening for cervical cancer involves the microscopic examination of cells scraped form the cervical os. This is a highly expensive and labour intensive process that is prone to failure. An alternative approach may be to screen for strains of the human papilloma virus that are closely linked to the development of malignancy and pilot studies have already begun (Manos *et al.*, 1999; Schoell *et al.*, 1999; Schneider, 1996). This can be readily carried out with existing technology and is likely to be less expensive and more accurate. However, undertaking the comparative trials needed to validate a new technique is likely to take a considerable length of time.

In patients with lung cancer, long-term survival depends critically on the stage of disease at diagnosis. Those with localised resectable disease have a much better outcome. In the past, screening tests using chest radiographs or sputum cytology have not proved effective at detecting early stage disease. However, recently there has been renewed interest in the possibility of screening heavy smokers with CT scanning or possibly molecular biological tests on sputum. Preliminary results suggest that this may be effective in detecting early resectable tumours before they produce symptoms. A screening programme of this type would be very expensive, particularly if expressed as the cost per life saved (Iwano *et al.*, 2000; Newman, 2000).

The main difference in screening practice will be an emphasis on identifying those at risk of development of cancer rather than the detection of early disease. It has long been recognised that some types of cancer have a strong familial tendency. Around 10 per cent of patients with breast cancer have a family history of the disease. Mutations of the gene BRCA1 are significantly more common in patients with early onset disease or a significant family history, than in the general population (Yang and Lippman, 1999; Coughlin *et al.*, 1999). It seems probable that BRCA1 is one of the growing family of tumour suppressor genes in which inactivation of both copies of the gene, by mutation or deletions, strongly predisposes to the development of cancer. If one abnormal copy of the gene is inherited it clearly much more likely that random genetic change will give rise to cells that have lost both copies and hence are at high risk of becoming malignant. Those who inherited a mutated BRCA 1 gene have a greatly increased lifetime risk of developing breast cancer. Studies have also shown that BRCA1 mutations are strongly associated with the development of ovarian cancer. Screening tests for BRCA1 mutations are now becoming available and may be marketed directly to the general public. Although there is still some doubt about the precise magnitude of the excess risk that can be attributed to BRCA1 mutations in healthy individuals, the management of those who have identified themselves as carriers by self-screening may soon become a common problem. The current options include intensive screening (Meiser *et al.*, 2000) or prophylactic bilateral mastectomy (Solomon *et al.*, 2000; Wagner *et al.*, 2000).

Colo-rectal carcinoma has also been shown to have a strong familial basis. Those with a family history of the disease have double the lifetime risk. This suggests that in most cases the inherited component is a relatively minor determinant of the condition. However, in about 5 per cent of cases genetic studies have shown a very strong dominant pattern of inheritance. This has been shown to be due to mutations in one of two genes. In hereditary non-polyposis colon cancer, the defective gene leads to failure to correct errors in DNA replication during cell division (Lynch, 1999). Those who inherit a mutated gene from one parent have a very high lifetime risk of developing colon cancer and women are also at risk of endometrial and ovarian cancer. The second inherited form of colon cancer is familial adenomatous polyposis. In this condition affected individuals develop very large number of colonic polyps with an almost 100 per cent risk that one or more of these benign tumours will become malignant (Allen, 1995; Ahnen, 1996; Potter, 1999).

Another important group of genes affecting cancer susceptibility are those that code for enzymes that are involved in the metabolism of external carcinogens, such as cigarette smoke. Many of these genes exist in several variant forms in the human population and the enzyme molecules produced differ in their level of activity. These variants have been shown to confer small but significant differences in risk of malignancy when exposed to environmental carcinogens such as cigarette smoke (Welfare *et al.*, 1999; Cheng *et al.*, 1999).

The completion of the 'human genome project' in the next few years will see an increasing catalogue of genes that alter an individual's susceptibility to a greater or lesser extent (Collins, 1999a; van Ommen *et al.*, 1999; Collins, 1999b). It is possible that the major application of this type of screening test will be outside the traditional healthcare setting, and that the central principle – that screening should only be carried out if there is a direct benefit to the patient – may no longer apply. Life insurance companies and employers may demand that prospective customers or employees are screened. Those deemed to be at risk may be severely disadvantaged in a number of important areas of their life and suffer considerable anxiety. It is relatively simple for an insurance company to assess risk in terms of cost of premiums and the effect on its business as a whole. It is extremely difficult for most individuals to make decisions on their own future based on the probability of a given event occurring in the future. This is made even more difficult where a subjective assessment of the seriousness of that event and the consequences of prophylactic intervention need to be considered. Helping well individuals who find themselves in this position will demand that nurses and others develop new skills in communication, assessment of risk and anxiety management. In many cases these decisions may be further complicated by the implications for other members of the family who may be similarly affected.

One consequence of the increasing ability to detect those at risk of developing cancer has been a growing interest in *chemoprevention* strategies. These involve the long-term treatment of healthy individuals with a drug that is designed to reduce the risk of development of a particular type of cancer. Clearly, it is essential the agents used in this way should have very low toxicity and be inexpensive. The design of clinical trials of chemoprevention necessarily involves very large numbers of individuals who must be followed up for many years. Individuals entered in these trials are selected because they have an excess risk, but even minor differences in how this group is defined may result in a different outcome of a trial and can make it difficult to compare results from different studies. This is seen in the use of tamoxifen to prevent breast cancer where a very positive outcome has been demonstrated in one large study but not repeated in smaller trials with slightly different entry criteria (Hong and Sporn, 1997; Decensi *et al.*, 2000; Minton, 2000). The importance of carrying out properly designed randomised trials is illustrated by the use of beta-carotene to prevent lung cancer in smokers. This is a natural compound with very low toxicity for which there were some theoretical reasons to predict a beneficial effect in preventing the development of lung cancer (Wright and Gruidl, 2000). However, trials actually showed an increased incidence of the disease in those treated.

Current Problems in Cancer Treatment

For most types of tumour, the best chance of a patient being cured of their disease lies in complete surgical excision. In general, the success of surgical treatment depends on early diagnosis. In most types of epithelial tumour, the probability of cure considerably decreases when local lymph nodes become involved. The presence of distant metastases generally indicates incurable disease, although in some cases resection of a solitary lung or hepatic tumour deposit may be beneficial.

Chemotherapy and radiotherapy alone or in combination are highly effective treatments for some types of leukaemia and lymphoma and for germ cell tumours. The success of these treatment protocols raises the question as to why chemotherapy and radiotherapy are much less effective as the sole treatment of the common epithelial malignancies. To answer this question requires a basic understanding of the mechanism of action of chemotherapy and radiotherapy.

The use of radiotherapy to treat malignant disease dates from the beginning of the twentieth century. Chemotherapy has its origin in the use of mustard gas during the First World War. In the context of what is now known about the molecular biology of the cancer cell, both chemotherapy and radiotherapy are relatively crude approaches to treatment. Radiotherapy and most types of chemotherapy act by causing damage to DNA. As the cell enters the cell cycle, prior to division, damage to DNA is detected and if the damage cannot be repaired the cell death programme is triggered and the cell dies (Ross, 1999b; Denmeade and Isaacs, 1996).

Two major factors limit this approach to therapy. First, these treatments are far from cancer cell specific and the tolerated dose will be set by toxicity to the bone marrow, the gastro-intestinal tract and other susceptible tissues. Second, many types of cancer cell are intrinsically resistant to the effects of chemotherapy and radiotherapy. The pathway by which DNA damage leads to cell death may be disrupted. One of the most common genetic abnormalities in epithelial tumours is mutation or deletion of the gene coding for the protein p53. This protein is a vital link between the system that detects DNA damage and the initiation of the cell death programme (King *et al.*, 1999; Blandino *et al.*, 1999). In other cells there may be inhibition of the cell death pathway itself through dysregulation of the control proteins. Tumour cells may also develop resistance to particular drugs through a variety of mechanisms. Amplification of the gene coding for the enzyme dihydrofolate reductase leads to resistance to methotrexate, which is a specific inhibitor of this enzyme. There may be a block in transport of anthracyclins to the nucleus or an increase in the activity of membrane pumps that reduce the effective intracellular drug concentration (Ogiso *et al.*, 2000; Wang and Cai, 1998; Berns *et al.*, 2000).

There are two basic strategies being investigated in an attempt to overcome these problems. First, techniques may be devised to protect normal tissues and allow higher doses of conventional chemotherapy to be given. Second, therapies can be devised that are specific to the cancer cell. The ultimate goal is to target the molecular abnormalities that distinguish the cancer cell from its normal counterparts and are responsible for the malignant behaviour of the cell.

Protecting Normal Tissues – the Use of Autologous Bone Marrow Transplantation

The ability of the bone marrow to continue to produce peripheral blood cells throughout life depends on a small number of stem cells (Golde, 1991). When these cells divide one of the daughter cells may become a progenitor cell. Progenitor cells pass through several rounds of cell division before all the cells produced differentiate into one of the cell types found in the peripheral blood – red cells, lymphocytes, etc. Stem cells have the critical property of being able to reconstitute the bone marrow when they are infused in sufficient numbers into a recipient whose marrow has been destroyed. To deliver chemotherapy in doses that would normally cause fatal marrow failure, the patient's bone marrow is harvested, stored and returned to the patient after completion of therapy. During the recovery phase after a dose of conventional chemotherapy, the administration of the bone marrow growth factor G-CSF will result in significant numbers of bone marrow stem cells and progenitor cells emerging into the peripheral blood. These cells can then be collected by cytophoresis. This procedure has almost completely replaced the collection of bone marrow by aspiration. The quality of the harvest is assessed by measuring the proportion of cells expressing the protein CD34 on their cell surface. This CD34 positive population is a mixture of stem cell and progenitor cells.

A major problem in using the patients own bone marrow cells is that the harvested cells may be contaminated by tumour cells that would be re-infused into the patient after chemotherapy. This is of particular concern in patients with lymphoma or myeloma where tumour involvement of the marrow is frequently present, although contamination may also occur with epithelial malignancy. Lymphoma cells often have a unique genetic fingerprint and highly sensitive PCR based techniques can be used to detect very low level of contamination of harvest samples. Although the evidence is relatively sparse, it appears that patients who receive a non-contaminated harvest may have a better outcome (Corradini *et al.*, 1999; Hardingham *et al.*, 1993; Freedman *et al.*, 2000). However, it is by no means certain that re-infusion of a small number of tumour cells will always lead to relapse. Various strategies are used to attempt to remove contaminating tumour cells from bone marrow. The most commonly used approach is to pass the harvested cells through a column of synthetic beads that are coated with a monoclonal antibody able to attach to CD34. This column will trap the CD34 expressing cells and progenitor cells, allowing the remaining cells, including any tumour cells to pass through. The attached cells can then be eluted and collected separately. This type of positive selection has the advantage in being potentially effective at removing any kind of tumour cell that does not express CD34. It is, however, very expensive and although it can be shown to be effective at reducing or eliminating contaminating tumour cells in many cases its value in improving patient outcomes has not yet been conclusively demonstrated (Fruehauf *et al.*, 1994; Freedman and Nadler, 1993).

The alternative approach to reducing marrow contamination is to attempt to destroy any tumour cells present in the harvest. This technique uses one or more monoclonal antibodies known to react to the patient's tumour cells. These are added to the harvest and in the presence of the complement proteins are able to destroy the tumour cells.

Allogenic transplantation, using donor marrow, may appear to be a solution to the problem of tumour cell contamination of harvests and it has been used to treat some patients with lymphoma and myeloma. However, in most studies the procedure related mortality outweighs any benefit compared to conventional therapy (Bierman, 2000) and is only applicable in those who have a suitable donor.

Although high dose therapy supported by autologous stem cell transplantation appears an attractive option, efficacy must be demonstrated in properly designed randomised clinical trials. Although the technique is now widely used in the treatment of haematological malignancy, a positive benefit has only been shown in a small number of trials and there is still uncertainty as the precise indications for this procedure (Simnett *et al.*, 2000). High dose therapy has also been widely used in the treatment of breast cancer. Patient demand resulted in this becoming a very common procedure in the United States in advance of any proven benefit (Bergh, 2000). Unfortunately, a number of major studies have now been reported showing that high dose therapy has no clear benefit for patients with breast cancer. This has two important lessons. First, simply increasing the dose of conventional chemotherapy does not necessarily increase its efficacy. This could have been predicted from the basic genetic abnormalities found in some tumour cells, as discussed above. Second, it is important to consider the factors that can create patient demand for a theoretically attractive but unproven therapy. The principle factor is almost certainly promotion of the technique in the media by enthusiastic proponents of the therapy. The theoretical basis for the treatment may sound plausible, or even self-evident, but experience has shown that a properly conducted clinical trial is the only acceptable demonstration of efficacy. As almost happened in the case of high dose therapy in breast cancer, the possibility of conducting trials may be subverted by patient demand possibly leading to an ineffective, hazardous and expensive procedure becoming the treatment of choice. Nurses have a key role in discussing with patients the importance of clinical trials and providing a balanced perspective on new therapeutic developments.

Increasing the Specificity of Treatment

A major goal in cancer therapy is to develop agents that target the tumour cell with the minimum damage to normal tissues. This has proved to be a very difficult problem as cancer cells have far more similarities to their normal counterpart than differences. However, a range of techniques are now being developed that make this goal more achievable in the coming years.

Monoclonal Antibody Therapy

Specific monoclonal antibodies can be made against almost any protein making them potentially useful as specific anti-tumour agents.

Monoclonal antibodies are usually produced in mice. If directly injected into a human, they would evoke an immune response to the mouse protein that would quickly inactivate any therapeutic effect. This can now be largely overcome by grafting the antigen binding sites of the mouse monoclonal antibody, which determine specificity, to the constant region of a human antibody molecule. The effect of monoclonal antibodies on cells is complex. When the antibody has bound its target on the surface of the tumour cell, it activates the complement protein in the blood. The end effect of this is to punch holes in the cell membrane and activate the cell death programme. Some antibodies may also activate cytotoxic lympho-cytes with a similar effect. In cultured cells, the addition of a monoclonal antibody may substitute for cytokine binding to specific receptors leading to alteration in the behaviour of the cell. In some cases, powerful toxins or radio-isotopes are attached to the antibody, which is used primarily as a means of delivering the active agent to the tumour cell. It should be noted that the specificity of these agents does not mean that they are entirely free of toxic effects.

Several therapeutic monoclonal antibodies are being used in clinical trials. None are tumour cell specific, but destroy the tumour cells and a restricted range of normal cells. The most widely used product is Rituximab. This targets CD20, a protein found on the surface of normal B-lymphocytes and many types of B-cell lymphoma. Numerous studies are underway to test the efficacy of this product in various types of lymphomas, either as a single agent or in combination with conventional chemotherapy (McLaughlin *et al.*, 1998; Maloney *et al.*, 1997). When this product was launched, it was widely reported in the press as a 'magic bullet' for cancer. This has generated patient demand for a product that is both very expensive and does not yet have a fully defined clinical role.

The human epidermal growth factor receptor 2 (HER2) is often expressed at high levels in breast cancer cells. Tumours that express this molecule tend to be more aggressive. Recently, a therapeutic antibody directed against HER2 has become available and early studies suggest that it make have a significant clinical effect in some patients. As is the case with Rituximab, it is possible that this agent may be most effective in combination with conventional cytotoxic drugs (Burris, 2000; Weiner, 1999; Dowsett *et al.*, 2000).

There are two potential limitations with antibody therapy. First, tumour cells often show great variability of expression of potential target molecules. Consequently, they may not be equally sensitive to the effects of the antibody. Second, further genetic change in the tumour cells may generate resistant clones that do not express the target molecule. Finally, effective monoclonal antibodies are currently very expensive.

Immunotherapy

A very influential idea in cancer research is the immune surveillance hypothesis. This proposes that a function of the normal immune system is to continually seek out and destroy cancer cells. It is failure of this system that allows clinically apparent tumours to develop. There is virtually no evidence that this theory is true, except possibly in a number of experimental animal tumours. However, the idea of using the very high levels of specificity of the immune system to target tumour cells has proved very attractive to many investigators. Even if anti-tumour surveillance is not a normal function of the immune system, it may be possible to induce an immunological attack on the tumour.

The starting point of the immune response is the processing of the antigenic molecule by dendritic cells. Foreign proteins are ingested by these cells, degraded into small peptides, some of which are then displayed on the cell surface attached to the HLA histocompatibility molecules. If a T-lymphocyte has a specific receptor able to bind to this molecular complex, and certain other conditions are fulfilled, this initiates an immune response. It is now possible to harvest dendritic cells from a patient's peripheral blood and maintain these in short term culture (Bubenik, 1999; Schreurs *et al.*, 2000; Hart and Hill, 1999). These cells can then be loaded with tumour related proteins in the hope that they will be displayed in a form that can be recognised by T-lymphocytes and will induce an anti-tumour immune response. These primed dendritic cells are then returned to the patient. There is anecdotal evidence and small studies that suggest that this technique can induce remission of a variety of types of tumour. One problem with this type of study is that ethical considerations often mean that the patients who are studied have failed to respond to multiple types of conventional therapy and are at an advanced stage of their disease. This may not be the optimal situation in which to test novel treatments of this type.

A special case of an anti-tumour immune response occurs in those receiving allogenic bone marrow transplantation. This technique, using cells donated by a sibling or an unrelated donor, is used mainly for the treatment of primary bone marrow malignancy where the tumour cells are derived from bone marrow stem cells or progenitor cells. These conditions include acute myeloid and lymphoblastic leukaemia, chronic myeloid leukaemia and myelodysplastic syndrome. One of the major problems of allogenic transplantation is the development of graft versus host disease. In this condition, T-lymphocytes from the donor attempt to reject the recipient as a foreign graft. This can produce severe skin, lung and gastro-intestinal problems and in some cases is fatal (Vogelsang, 2000). A solution to this problem is to remove the T-lymphocytes from the graft, using monoclonal antibodies, before transplantation. This abolishes graft versus host disease but unfortunately produces a much higher rate of relapse. This led to the realisation that the donor lymphocytes were also exerting a very import-ant graft versus leukaemia effect in destroying a small number of residual leukaemia cells that had survived the conditioning radiotherapy or chemo-therapy (Appelbaum, 1997). Many studies are now underway into this effect and how it can be manipulated to prevent graft versus host disease, but maximise the anti-leukaemia effect. T-lymphocytes can be separated from the bone marrow harvest and stored. These cells can then be re-infused in controlled doses at intervals after the transplant to maximise the anti-leukaemic effect while minimising the graft versus host reaction. In chronic myeloid leukaemia, molecular monitoring techniques can be used to detect evidence of relapse far below the stage of clinically detectable disease. In many of these patients remission can be re-established using infusions of donor lymphocytes (Porter *et al.*, 1999; du and Novitzky, 1999).

A further development of this technology is the mini-allogenic trans-plant. This technique aims to optimise the potential benefits to patients without the hazards of full myelo-ablative chemotherapy, allowing the technique to be used in a broader group of patients. The patient is given a less intensive form of conditioning chemotherapy, sufficient to allow the donor marrow to engraft but without necessarily completely destroying the patient's own marrow. This allows donor lymphocytes to be given in an attempt to destroy residual tumour cells. Clinical trials of this technique are at an early stage (Carella *et al.*, 2000). There are many unanswered questions as to the cellular mechanism of the donor lymphocyte anti-tumour effect and which types of tumour are likely to be responsive to this approach.

Targeting the Genetic Defects in the Tumour Cells

The ideal target for specific therapy would be the genetic abnormalities present in the cancer cell that are responsible for its malignant behaviour. Retinoic acid is essential to the differentiation of a range of cell types. In the bone marrow, retinoic acid is required for the differentiation of progenitor cells to form granulocytes. In acute promyelocytic leukaemia a chromosomal translocation, involving one of the genes coding for the receptor through which retinoic acid acts, renders the cell insensitive to retinoic acid and cellular differentiation is blocked. This can be overcome using high doses of all trans retinoic acid (ATRA). This causes the leukaemic blast cells to differentiate to mature granulocytes within a few days of starting treatment. Granulocytes do not divide and die after a short interval. This is now the standard initial therapy for acute promyelocytic leukaemia (Mandelli, 1997).

Recently, targeted chemotherapy has become available for patients with chronic myeloid leukaemia (CML). CML has a specific chromosomal translocation which produces a novel cellular enzyme, *bcr – abl*. This protein has a key role in the development of leukaemia. Knowledge of the structure of this protein has been used to produce a specific inhibitor – *STI571* (Goldman, 2000). Early clinical trials suggest that this is a highly effective agent for this condition, for which allogenic bone marrow transplantation is currently the only potentially curative treatment. This is likely to be the first of many novel agents produced as a result of rational drug design based on knowledge of the molecular biology of the cancer cell.

An alternative approach is to attempt to block the expression of genes that are aberrantly expressed in the tumour cells. One approach is to use anti-sense oligonucleotides. Gene expression involves making an RNA copy of the coding of the DNA sequence. This molecule is transported to the cell cytoplasm and translated into protein. The addition of an RNA sequence that is complementary to the messenger RNA results in the formation of a double stranded molecule that is rapidly degraded, blocking protein synthesis. Although this is conceptually attractive, there are major problems in putting this into practice. First, the anti-sense molecule must be delivered to the tumour cells in an active form. Second, it has been found that some anti-sense molecules may be toxic through pharmacological properties independent of their specific effect. Third, blocking a specific gene – unless it results in cell death – may be a transient effect. Despite these problems, several clinical trials of antisense therapy are now underway (Clark, 2000; Cotter, 1999; Warzocha, 1999).

A highly innovative approach to specific therapy is to use defective viruses to lyse the tumour cells. Normal adenovirus causes a 'common cold' like illness. The virus enters cells and replicates itself. The cell is either ruptured releasing the virus, or is destroyed by the immune system. To complete this cycle, the virus must inhibit the function of the infected cell's *p53* protein. A defective virus has been produced that can no longer inhibit *p53* and so is incapable of replication in normal cells. However, the virus can replicate itself in tumour cells where *p53* has been inactivated (Gurnani *et al.*, 1999; Lowe, 1999). As each tumour cell is destroyed, it produces sufficient virus to infect several others. Trials of this anti-tumour virus therapy are being carried out in head and neck cancer (Gurnani *et al.*, 1999).

Gene Therapy

In the longer term it is possible that genetic modification of cells may play a major role in cancer therapy. The DNA sequence for a particular gene can be cloned and joined to other sequences that are known to regulate gene expression. This artificial construct is then inserted into a cell where, hopefully, it will become integrated into a host chromosome, and the gene will begin to be expressed. In theory, this technology could be used to replace dysfunctional genes in tumour cells, although there are major problems to be overcome. One of the most difficult of these problems is to design a method of packaging the cloned DNA to ensure that it is delivered efficiently to the target cell. A favoured method is to use modified viruses to carry the novel genetic material in the cell. However, there are important safety considerations to be met before releasing genetically modified viruses into the general environment (Aspinall and Lemoine, 1999; Anderson, 2000).

Despite these problems, there are several genetic manipulation techniques already at the stage of early clinical trial. The easiest targets for genetic manipulation are harvest bone marrow cells before they are returned to the patient. Bone marrow harvest cells can be transfected with genes coding for proteins that increase the resistance to chemotherapy (Brenner, 1999; Rosenberg *et al.*, 2000). After transplant, the bone marrow will be more resistant to any subsequent chemotherapy. Another approach is to attempt to produce DNA vaccines to the tumour cells. If a cloned DNA sequence – coding for a tumour specific protein – is injected intramuscularly, some of the DNA is taken up by the muscle cells which then produce the protein. In this context, the protein may be recognised as foreign by the immune system and an immune response initiated. This may result in the destruction of the tumour cells that express the protein. DNA vaccines are currently being developed for the treatment of some types of lymphoma (Kwak, 1998).

Targeting the Tumour Stroma

It is increasingly recognised that tumour cells are far from autonomous and depend on surrounding normal cells. These cells, known collectively as stromal cells, may provide anchorage for the tumour cells or secrete important growth factors or survival signals that the tumour cells require. The ability to stimulate new blood vessel formation is a key element in the development of many types of tumour. As the tumour grows, vessels are required to carry oxygen and other nutrients to the centre of the tumour. The tendency to form metastatic deposits is increased in highly vascularised tumours. A range of new drugs have been developed to attempt to inhibit new blood vessel formation in tumours. Experimental evidence suggests that that these may be highly synergistic with anti-tumour chemotherapy. These agents are now being used in clinical trials. Although the clinical studies are in their infancy, an important new concept arising from this work is that successful therapy may depend on targeting both the cancer cell and its supporting normal cells (Harris, 1997; Hui and Ignoffo, 1998; Eckhardt, 1999).

Implications for Practice

One of the aims of this chapter was to show that the next decade is going to be a period of very rapid change in oncology. Nurses working in this field will find themselves faced with a range of challenges. The delivery of some types of treatment may be technically demanding and possibly associated with novel short and long-term toxicity. Patients who are incurable by conventional therapy may increasingly be recruited into pilot studies of new agents raising potential ethical problems in balancing the possible benefits to the patients and the importance of the trial against conventional palliative care protocols.

However, it is the changes in the social context in which cancer care is delivered that may give rise to the most difficult problems for nurses and other healthcare professionals. The volume of information freely available to many patients has already increased dramatically and this trend will accelerate. Cancer is a very frequent topic in all newspapers and on television and the number of cancer related sites on the internet is already enormous. Nurses are now only one of many sources of information. It must be remembered that the media is commercially driven and has little obligation to explain complex concepts. Pharmaceutical and other interests have large investments in oncology related areas and can promote their products directly to patient through media management and possibly soon by direct advertising. It is important that nurses are able to help the patient to form an accurate and balanced view of the relevant issues. This may be particularly difficult where a novel therapy, that appears to offer hope to the patient, is being promoted without reliable evidence of efficacy. A more difficult situation may be where a treatment has been shown to be of proven efficacy but is not provided on the basis of cost.

It is very unlikely that healthcare professionals will continue to have control over access to genetic screening. Individuals will be able, through commercial laboratories, to obtain information on their own genetic characteristics. This may be undertaken freely or at the request of a third party. The problem will not be a patient with cancer but a person, or possibly an entire family, with a defined risk of developing the disease. At present there are few nurses who possess the skills required to help individuals in this situation come to reasonable decisions. These decisions are potentially much more complex than assessing the relative merits of the various treatment options of someone who already has cancer.

The increasing specialisation of cancer care has directly influenced nursing. There are large numbers of specialist nurses working in cancer and palliative care, in cancer screening, in genetic services, in cancer research and education. In the United Kingdom, this growth of new roles for nurses has led to some confusion. Working as a specialist practitioner (UKCC, 1994) has become confused with the role of clinical nurse specialist and nurse practitioner (UKCC, 1999). Current initiatives to provide clear descriptors for 'higher level practice' and the new 'nurse consultant' role (DOH, 1999; UKCC, 2002) should provide a career framework that is transparent while protecting the public through professional standards.

Finally, it is important that nurse educators recognise the importance of a basic understanding of the principles of cellular biology and biotechnology. These ideas will touch almost every aspect of healthcare in the coming years. Without this, knowledge nurses will be ill equipped to provide effective care for their patients.

References

Ahnen, D.J. (1996) The genetic basis of colorectal cancer risk. *Advances in Internal Medicine*, 41, 531–52.

Allen, J.I. (1995) Molecular biology of colon polyps and colon cancer. *Seminars in Surgical Oncology*, 11, 399–405.

Anderson, W.F. (2000) Gene therapy. The best of times, the worst of times [comment]. *Science*, 288, 627–9.

Appelbaum, F.R. (1997) Graft versus leukemia (GVL) in the therapy of acute lymphoblastic leukemia (ALL). *Leukemia*, 11, Suppl. 4, S15–7.

Aspinall, R.J. and N.R. Lemoine (1999) Gene therapy for pancreatic and biliary malignancies. *Annals of Oncology*, 10, Suppl. 4, 188–92.

Bergh, J. (2000) Where next with stem-cell-supported high-dose therapy for breast cancer? [comment]. *Lancet*, 355, 944–5.

Berns, E.M., J.A. Foekens, R. Vossen, M.P. Look, P. Devilee, S.C. Henzen-Logmans, I.L. van Staveren, W.L. van Putten, M. Inganas, M.E. Meijer-van Gelder, C. Cornelisse, C.J. Claassen, H. Portengen, B. Bakker and J.G. Klijn (2000) Complete sequencing of TP53 predicts poor response to systemic therapy of advanced breast cancer. *Cancer Reserch*, 60, 2155–62.

Berrino, F., G. Gatta, E. Chessa, F. Valente and R. Capocaccia (1998) The EUROCARE II study. *European Journal of Cancer*, 34, 2139–53.

Bierman, P.J. (2000) Allogeneic bone marrow transplantation for lymphoma [In Process Citation]. *Blood Review*, 14, 1–13.

Bishop, J.M. (1982) Oncogenes. *Scientific American*, 246, 80–92.

Blandino, G., A.J. Levine and M. Oren (1999) Mutant *p53* gain of function: differential effects of different *p53* mutants on resistance of cultured cells to chemotherapy. *Oncogene*, 18, 477–85.

Brenner, M. (1999) Resistance is futile [comment]. *Gene Therapy*, 6, 1646–7.

Bubenik, J. (1999) Dendritic-cell-based cancer vaccines [editorial]. *Folia Biol.(Praha)*, 45, 71–4.

Burris III, H.A. (2000) Docetaxel (Taxotere) in HER-2-positive patients and in combination with trastuzumab (Herceptin) [In Process Citation]. *Seminars in Oncology*, 27, 19–23.

Butel, J.S. (2000) Viral carcinogenesis: revelation of molecular mechanisms and etiology of human disease. *Carcinogenesis*, 21, 405–26.

Carella, A.M., R. Champlin, S. Slavin, P. McSweeney and R. Storb (2000) Mini-allografts: ongoing trials in humans [editorial]. *Bone Marrow Transplant*, 25, 345–50.

Chen, P.M., T.J. Chiou, R.K. Hsieh, F.S. Fan, C.J. Chu, C.Z. Lin, H. Chiang, C.C. Yen, W.S. Wang and J.H. Liu (1999) *p53* gene mutations and rearrangements in non-Hodgkin's lymphoma. *Cancer*, 85, 718–24.

Cheng, L., E.M. Sturgis, S.A. Eicher, D. Char, M.R. Spitz and Q. Wei (1999) Glutathione-S-transferase polymorphisms and risk of squamous-cell carcinoma of the head and neck. *International Journal of Cancer*, 84, 220–24.

Clark, R.E. (2000) Antisense therapeutics in chronic myeloid leukaemia: the promise, the progress and the problems. *Leukemia*, 14, 347–55.

Collins, F.S. (1999a) Genetics: an explosion of knowledge is transforming clinical practice. *Geriatrics*, 54, 41–7.

Collins, F.S. (1999b) The human genome project and the future of medicine. *Annals of the New York Academy of Science*, 882, 42–55.

Corradini, P., M. Ladetto, A. Pileri and C. Tarella (1999) Clinical relevance of minimal residual disease monitoring in non- Hodgkin's lymphomas: a critical reappraisal of molecular strategies. *Leukemia*, 13, 1691–5.

Cotter, F.E. (1999) Antisense therapy of hematologic malignancies. *Seminars in Hematology*, 36, 9–14.

Coughlin, S.S., M.J. Khoury and K.K. Steinberg (1999) BRCA1 and BRCA2 gene mutations and risk of breast cancer. Public health perspectives. *American Journal of Preventative Medicine*, 16, 91–8.

Decensi, A., B. Bonanni, A. Guerrieri-Gonzaga, R. Torrisi, L. Manetti, C. Robertson, G. De Palo, F. Formelli, A. Costa and U. Veronesi (2000) Chemoprevention of breast cancer: the Italian experience [In Process Citation]. *Journal of Cell Biochemistry*, Suppl, 34, 84–96.

Denmeade, S.R. and J.T. Isaacs (1996) Programmed Cell Death (Apoptosis) and Cancer Chemotherapy. *Cancer Control*, 3, 303–9.

Department of Health (1999) *Making a Difference*. London: Department of Health.

Dowsett, M., T. Cooke, I. Ellis, W.J. Gullick, B. Gusterson, E. Mallon and R. Walker (2000) Assessment of HER2 status in breast cancer: why, when and how? *European Journal of Cancer*, 36, 170–6.

du, T.C. and N. Novitzky (1999) GVL and GVHD following the infusion of a limited number of donor CD3 cells in the therapy of leukaemia relapse after bone marrow transplantation [letter]. *European Journal of Haematology*, 62, 68–9.

Eckhardt, S.G. (1999) Angiogenesis inhibitors as cancer therapy. *Hospital Practice*, 34, 63–9, 83.

Erickson, D. (1990) Of mice and men. How form affects function in monoclonal-antibody drugs. *Scientific American*, 262, 76–7.

Freedman, A., J.W. Friedberg and J. Gribben (2000) High-dose therapy for follicular lymphoma. *Oncology*, 14, 321–6, 329.

Freedman, A.S. and L.M. Nadler (1993) Developments in purging in autotransplantation. [Review]. *Hematology – Oncology Clinics of North America*, 7, 687–715.

Fruehauf, S., R. Haas, W.J. Zeller and W. Hunstein (1994) CD34 selection for purging in multiple myeloma and analysis of CD34 + B cell precursors. *Stem Cells*, 12, 95–102.

Golde, D.W. (1991) The stem cell. *Scientific American*, 265, 86–93.

Goldman, J.M. (2000) Tyrosine-kinase inhibition in treatment of chronic myeloid leukaemia. *Lancet*, 355, 1031–2.

Greaves, M.F., W. Verbi, R. Tilley, T.A. Lister, J. Habeshaw, H.G. Guo, C.D. Trainor, M. Robert-Guroff, W. Blattner and M. Reitz (1984) Human T-cell leukemia virus (HTLV) in the United Kingdom. *Internationl Journal of Cancer*, 33, 795–806.

Gurnani, M., P. Lipari, J. Dell, B. Shi and L.L. Nielsen (1999) Adenovirus-mediated *p53* gene therapy has greater efficacy when combined with chemotherapy against human head and neck, ovarian, prostate, and breast cancer. *Cancer Chemotherapy & Pharmacology*, 44, 143–51.

Hardingham, J.E., D. Kotasek, R.E. Sage, A. Dobrovic, T. Gooley and B.M. Dale (1993) Molecular detection of residual lymphoma cells in peripheral blood stem cell harvests and following autologous transplantation. *Bone Marrow Transplantation*, 11, 15–20.

Harris, A.L. (1997) Antiangiogenesis for cancer therapy. *Lancet*, 349, Suppl. 2, SII13–15.

Hart, D.N. and G.R. Hill (1999) Dendritic cell immunotherapy for cancer: application to low-grade lymphoma and multiple myeloma. *Immunology & Cell Biology*, 77, 451–9.

Henn, W. (1999) Genetic screening with the DNA chip: a new Pandora's box? *Journal of Medical Ethics*, 25, 200–3.

Hong, W.K. and M.B. Sporn (1997) Recent advances in chemoprevention of cancer. *Science*, 278, 1073–7.

Hui, Y.F. and R.J. Ignoffo (1998) Angiogenesis inhibitors. A promising role in cancer therapy. *Cancer Practice*, 6, 60–2.

Iwano, S., N. Makino, M. Ikeda, S. Itoh, S. Ishihara, M. Tadokoro and T. Ishigaki (2000) Video-taped helical CT images for lung cancer screening. *Journal of Computer Assisted Tomography*, 24, 242–6.

Jurcic, J.G., D.A. Scheinberg and A.N. Houghton (1997) Monoclonal antibody therapy of cancer. *Cancer Chemotherapy & Biological Response Modification*, 17, 195–216.

King, T.C., O.C. Estalilla and H. Safran (1999) Role of *p53* and *p16* gene alterations in determining response to concurrent paclitaxel and radiation in solid tumor. *Seminars in Radiation Oncology*, 9, 4–11.

Kinoshita, J. (1990) The oncogene connection. *Scientific American*, 262, 24, 24D.

Komiya, T., T. Hirashima and I. Kawase (1999) Clinical significance of *p53* in non-small-cell lung cancer. *Oncology Reports*, 6, 19–28.

Kurian, K.M., C.J. Watson and A.H. Wyllie (1999) DNA chip technology. *Journal of Pathology*, 187, 267–71.

Kwak, L.W. (1998) Tumor vaccination strategies combined with autologous peripheral stem cell transplantation. *Annals of Oncology*, 9, Suppl. 1, S41–46.

Link, B.K. and G.J. Weiner (1998) Monoclonal antibodies in the treatment of human B-cell malignancies. *Leukaemia & Lymphoma*, 31, 237–49.

Lowe, S.W. (1999) Activation of p53 by oncogenes. *Endocrine Related Cancer*, 6, 45–8.

Lundberg, A.S. and R.A. Weinberg (1999) Control of the cell cycle and apoptosis. *European Journal of Cancer*, 35, 1886–94.

Lynch, H.T. (1999) Hereditary nonpolyposis colorectal cancer (HNPCC). *Cytogenetic Cell Genetics*, 86, 130–5.

Madhukar, B.V. and J.E. Trosko (1997) The causes of cancer: implications for prevention and treatment. *Indian Journal of Pediatrics*, 64, 131–41.

Maloney, D.G., A.J. Grillo-Lopez, C.A. White, D. Bodkin, R.J. Schilder, J.A. Neidhart, N. Janakira-man, K.A. Foon, T.M. Liles, B.K. Dallaire, K. Wey, I. Royston, T. Davis and R. Levy (1997) IDEC-C2B8 (Rituximab) anti-CD20 monoclonal antibody therapy in patients with relapsed low-grade non-Hodgkin's lymphoma. *Blood*, 90, 2188–95.

Mandelli, F. (1997) New strategies for the treatment of acute promyelocytic leukaemia. *Journal of Internal Medicine*, Suppl, 740, 23–7.

Manns, A., M. Hisada and L. La Grenade (1999) Human T-lymphotropic virus type I infection. *Lancet*, 353, 1951–8.

Manos, M.M., W.K. Kinney, L.B. Hurley, M.E. Sherman, J. Shieh-Ngai, R.J. Kurman, J.E. Ransley, B.J. Fetterman, J.S. Hartinger, K.M. McIntosh, G.F. Pawlick and R.A. Hiatt (1999) Identifying women with cervical neoplasia: using human papillomavirus DNA testing for equivocal Papanicolaou results. *Journal of the American Medical Association*, 281, 1605–10.

McLaughlin, P., A.J. Grillo-Lopez, B.K. Link, R. Levy, M.S. Czuczman, M.E. Williams, M.R. Heyman, I. Bence-Bruckler, C.A. White, F. Cabanillas, V. Jain, A.D. Ho, J. Lister, K. Wey, D. Shen and B.K. Dallaire (1998) Rituximab chimeric anti-CD20 monoclonal antibody therapy for relapsed indolent lymphoma: half of patients respond to a four-dose treatment program. *Journal of Clinical Oncology*, 16, 2825–33.

Meijerink, J.P. (1997) t(14;18), a journey to eternity. *Leukemia*, 11, 2175–87.

Meiser, B., P. Butow, A. Barratt, M. Friedlander, J. Kirk, C. Gaff, E. Haan, K. Aittomaki and K. Tucker (2000) Breast cancer screening uptake in women at increased risk of developing hereditary breast cancer [In Process Citation]. *Breast Cancer Research & Treatment*, 59, 101–11.

Milstein, C. (1980) Monoclonal antibodies. *Scientific American*, 243, 66–74.

Minton, S.E. (2000) Chemoprevention of breast cancer in the older patient. *Hematological & Oncological Clinics of North America*, 14, 113–30.

Mullis, K.B. (1990) The unusual origin of the polymerase chain reaction. *Scientific American*, 262, 56–65.

Newman, L. (2000) Larger debate underlies spiral CT screening for lung cancer [In Process Citation]. *Journal of the National Cancer Institute*, 92, 592–4.

Ogawa, Y., A. Nishioka, T. Inomata, T. Ohnishi, S. Kariya, M. Terashima, S. Yoshida, N. Tohchika, Y. Tanaka and M. Kumon (2000) Conservation treatment intensified with an anti-estrogen agent and CAF chemotherapy for stage I and II breast cancer [In Process Citation]. *Oncology Report*, 7, 479–84.

Ogiso, Y., A. Tomida, S. Lei, S. Omura and T. Tsuruo (2000) Proteasome inhibition circumvents solid tumor resistance to topoisomerase II-directed drugs [In Process Citation]. *Cancer Research*, 60, 2429–34.

Park, C.C., M. Mitsumori, A. Nixon, A. Recht, J. Connolly, R. Gelman, B. Silver, S. Hetelekidis, A. Abner, J.R. Harris and S.J. Schnitt (2000) Outcome at 8 years after breast-conserving surgery and radiation therapy for invasive breast cancer: influence of margin status and systemic therapy on local recurrence [in process citation]. *Journal of Clinical Oncology*, 18, 1668–75.

Pincus, M.R., P.W. Brandt-Rauf, J. Michl, R.P. Carty and F.K. Friedman (2000) ras-p21-induced cell transformation: unique signal transduction pathways and implications for the design of new chemotherapeutic agents. *Cancer Investigation*, 18, 39–50.

Porter, D.L., R.H. Collins, Jr, O. Shpilberg, W.R. Drobyski, J.M. Connors, A. Sproles and J.H. Antin (1999) Long-term follow-up of patients who achieved complete remission after donor leukocyte infusions. *Biol. Blood Marrow Transplant*, 5, 253–61.

Potter, J.D. (1999) Colorectal cancer: molecules and populations. *Journal of the National Cancer Institute*, 91, 916–32.

Rosenberg, S.A., R.M. Blaese, M.K. Brenner, A.B. Deisseroth, F.D. Ledley, M.T. Lotze, J.M. Wilson, G.J. Nabel, K. Cornetta, J.S. Economou, S.M. Freeman, S.R. Riddell, M. Brenner, E. Oldfield, B. Gansbacher, C. Dunbar, R.E. Walker, F.G. Schuening, J.A. Roth, R.G. Crystal, M.J. Welsh, K. Culver, H.E. Heslop, J. Simons, R.W. Wilmott and R.C. Boucher (2000) Human gene marker/ therapy clinical protocols [In Process Citation]. *Human Gene Therapy*, 11, 919–79.

Ross, G.M. (1999) Induction of cell death by radiotherapy. *Endocrine Related Cancer*, 6, 41–4.

Schneider, A. (1996) Virologic screening. *European Journal of Obstetrics Gynecology & Reproductive Biology*, 65, 61–3.

Schoell, W.M., M.F. Janicek and R. Mirhashemi (1999) Epidemiology and biology of cervical cancer. *Seminars in Surgical Oncology*, 16, 203–11.

Schreurs, M.W., A.A. Eggert, C.J. Punt, C.G. Figdor and G.J. Adema (2000) Dendritic cell-based vaccines: from mouse models to clinical cancer immunotherapy [In Process Citation]. *Critical Reviews in Oncology*, 11, 1–17.

Simnett, S.J., L.A. Stewart, J. Sweetenham, G. Morgan and P.W. Johnson (2000) Autologous stem cell transplantation for malignancy: a systematic review of the literature. *Clinical Laboratory Haematology*, 22, 61–72.

Solomon, J.S., C.F. Brunicardi and J.D. Friedman (2000) Evaluation and treatment of BRCA-positive patients. *Plastic Reconstructive Surgery*, 105, 714–19.

Tarapore, P. and K. Fukasawa (2000) p53 mutation and mitotic infidelity. *Cancer Investigation*, 18, 148–55.

Tokino, T. and Y. Nakamura (2000) The role of p53-target genes in human cancer. *Critical Reviews in Oncology & Hematology*, 33, 1–6.

UKCC (1994) *The Future of Professional Practice: the Council's Standards for Education and Practice Following Registration*. London: UKCC.

UKCC (1999) *A Higher Level of Practice*. London: UKCC.

UKCC (2002) *Report of the Higher Level Practice Pilot and Project*. London: UKCC.

Vaandrager, J.W., E. Schuuring, T. Raap, K. Philippo, K. Kleiverda and P. Kluin (2000) Interphase FISH detection of BCL2 rearrangement in follicular lymphoma using breakpoint-flanking probes. *Genes Chromosomes Cancer*, 27, 85–94.

van Ommen, G.J., E. Bakker and J.T. den Dunnen (1999) The human genome project and the future of diagnostics, treatment, and prevention [In Process Citation]. *Lancet*, 354 Suppl. 1, SI5–10.

Vogelsang, G.B. (2000) Advances in the treatment of graft-versus-host disease. *Leukemia*, 14, 509–10.

Wagner, H.P. (1998) Cell cycle control and cancer. *Indian Journal of Pediatrics*, 65, 805–14.

Wagner, T.M., R. Moslinger, G. Langbauer, R. Ahner, E. Fleischmann, A. Auterith, A. Friedmann, T. Helbich, C. Zielinski, E. Pittermann, M. Seifert and P. Oefner (2000) Attitude towards prophylactic surgery and effects of genetic counselling in families with BRCA mutations. Austrian Hereditary Breast and Ovarian Cancer Group. *British Journal Cancer*, 82, 1249–53.

Wallace, R.W. (1997) DNA on a chip: serving up the genome for diagnostics and research. *Molecular Medical Today*, 3, 384–9.

Wang, S. and G. Cai (1998) Clinical study of multi-drug resistance gene (MDR1) expression in primary ovarian cancer [In Process Citation]. *Journal of Tongji Medical University*, 18, 58–60.

Warzocha, K. (1999) Antisense strategy in hematological malignancies. *Cytokines Cell Molecular Therapy*, 5, 15–23.

Weinberg, R.A. (1983) A molecular basis of cancer. *Scientific American*, 249, 126–42.

Weinberg, R.A. (1996) How cancer arises. *Scientific American*, 275, 62–70.

Weiner, L.M. (1999) Monoclonal antibody therapy of cancer. *Seminars in Oncology*, 26, 43–51.

Welfare, M., A.A. Monesola, M.F. Bassendine and A.K. Daly (1999) Polymorphisms in GSTP1, GSTM1, and GSTT1 and susceptibility to colorectal cancer. *Cancer & Epidemiology. Biomarkers Prevention*, 8, 289–92.

Wright, G.S. and M.E. Gruidl (2000) Early detection and prevention of lung cancer. *Current Opinion in Oncology*, 12, 143–8.

Yang, X. and M.E. Lippman (1999) BRCA1 and BRCA2 in breast cancer. *Breast Cancer Research & Treatment*, 54, 1–10.

6

Advancing Practice in Family Nursing Across the Cancer Continuum

JEAN FLANAGAN, SUSAN HOLMES and DOUG MCINNES

Introduction

It has been observed that cancer is a 'family disease' (Costain-Schou and Hewison, 1999). Certainly the family, or significant others in the support network are critical to the psychological well-being and adaptation of the person with cancer (Carlsson and Hamrin, 1994; Dunkel-Schetter *et al.*, 1992). Conversely the literature is replete with examples of the impact of cancer on the family and much focused work has been undertaken to identify their unique needs, as distinct from the needs of the individual with cancer. Yet family care is considered by many to be a neglected area in nursing practice (Plant 1995; Whyte and Robb, 1999). Working with families is complex and demanding work and requires a high level of skill from the practitioner; however, there is enormous potential for role expansion and role development. A family centred approach to care is suggested as a means by which practice can be improved. It is the intention here to critically examine the very differing theoretical perspectives of 'family centred care' in order that practitioners can assess for themselves the utility and validity of strategies and techniques to harness the potential of the family or personal/ social network in their care of the person with cancer.

What is 'The Family' in Family Centred Care?

A central tenet of the family nursing movement is a shift from viewing the individual as the unit of care to incorporating key 'family members' in nursing care. Conceptually 'the family' is defined very broadly in most theoretical definitions of family nursing which aggregate dissimilar concepts. One of the very real issues which family nursing must face is the changing nature of contemporary households. Indeed, most social science analysts have long since abandoned traditional notions of 'the family' and replaced these with the concept of the household. In a society of mobility, social dynamism, divorce, diverse and multivarious personal relationships, old ideas of the family seem much less relevant to modern society. The extended family model and even the nuclear family model have been abandoned, and this is reflected in the numbers that are clearly apparent from social statistics and social indicators.

Most contemporary theoretical definitions of family nursing, or family care, have a broad definition of the family, which incorporate different family forms. For example, defining family as 'two or more people joined together by bonds of sharing or intimacy' (Baider and De Nour, 1994). Family can also be defined by its functions. A family thus: provides for the physical and health needs of its members serves as a locus of love, intimacy and motivation provides sociologic and psychologic roots (Baider and De Nour, 1994).

While for practical purposes the most relevant definition may be that 'the family is who the patients says it is', this definition is likely to be too vague to those undertaking research where the definition has implications for sampling and measurement (McClement and Woodgate, 1998). Concepts of 'family in family nursing' may well be a misnomer, since in most cases it is the patient's whole social network that is being considered rather than a specific form of domestic relationship. The body of knowledge from family nursing and social support thus supports this discussion. In the remainder of this discussion the term family will be used interchangeably with personal/social network.

Impact of the Family/Personal Social Network on Illness: Factors Influencing the Personal Social Network in Cancer and Palliative Care

Cancer patients typically experience an increased need for love, support and affection that may increase over the trajectory of the disease and treatments (Dunkel-Schetter *et al.*, 1992). However, fear of rejection and abandonment are frequent and accompany poor communication between patients, families and friends (Carlsson and Hamrin, 1994). This is partly a consequence of the public misconceptions of cancer being contagious and its associations with death which evokes excessive fear, anxiety and stigma, resulting in avoidance behaviour of families and friends (Fallow-field, 1990; Picardie, 1998; Peters-Golden, 1982; Wortman, 1984). Other factors in miscommunication may relate to pretence by family and friends through maintenance of a cheerful and optimistic outlook despite harbouring negative feelings about cancer. Krishnasamy (1996) argues that such contradictions cannot reassure individuals who may be highly fearful and uncertain. Unintentional avoidance behaviours can be damaging to the person with cancer as they can be viewed as rejection. This occurs at the very time when support from others is especially important (Dunkel-Schetter *et al.*, 1992). The social relationship has potential to work, as a psychological mediator following a cancer diagnosis and skilled nursing will harness this resource, rather than undermine it. It is essential therefore that all nurses working with those with cancer understand the importance of social relationship and how it works.

What is a Social Relationship, and How Does it Work?

The idea that social relationships influence well-being has been advocated by many theorists (Bowlby, 1969; Durkheim, 1981). The function of the relationship has been described as 'giving information to a loved one that he/she is cared for, valued and belongs to a mutually obliging communication network' (Cobb, 1976). The study of this social relationship has been conceptualised as the study of social support. Support may be expressed through social interactions, or through functional components, that is emotional, instrumental, or informational support with potential to buffer major life events (Wills, 1985). The literature is replete with examples of the benefits of social support and the detriments of its absence. An individual's satisfaction with perceived, or actual support, can influence the effectiveness of social support. This is demonstrated in a group study of cancer patients by Peters-Golden (1982) who revealed that patients assert that the support extended to them is often inappropriate in nature. Patients reported non-materialisation of expected support networks and decreased adjustment to the cancer diagnosis because of this experience. As a result of this and similar research findings social support researchers have sought to investigate the factors that determine when actions are supportive, or not, for someone who is suffering. The person providing the support may be an important variable, for example in a study of 79 cancer patients, Dunkel-Schetter (1984) found information and advice from physicians were seen as being helpful, but that these same behaviours were unhelpful when performed by family and friends. Her suggestions, from studies in the late 1970s, of a 'victimisation effect', with people with cancer experiencing rejection, withdrawal and communication problems, because of the stigma of cancer, has been challenged by Dakof and Taylor (1990). They suggest that the 'victimisation hypothesis' may be more pertinent to relationships that have few cultural constraints to keep parties involved with one another, for example friends or acquaintances. Not only may family members be committed to the relationship and unlikely to withdraw support, but also they may also be more likely to demonstrate over involvement or overprotective behaviours than withdrawal (Coyne *et al.*, 1998). Clearly there are multiple factors influencing quality in the social relationships of the person with a cancer diagnosis. Members of the support network, and close contacts in particular, have to manage the ill person's response to the illness and their own psychological reactions. The impact upon their psychological well-being can be profound, hence their needs and concerns, as family members, are therefore of concern to the cancer and palliative care nurse.

Impact of Life Threatening Illness on the Family: Responses and Needs of Families

Cancer disrupts the family and alters its expectations for the future. The family may move from a position of stability to instability that may be permanent. Several studies have heightened awareness of the negative impact of a cancer diagnosis upon the family. In an exploration of the ways in which people live with a diagnosis of cancer, Plant (1995) demonstrated differences between the family and patient, not only in their experience of the illness but also in their perceptions and reactions to it. This creates an additional burden on both parties as the patient and family live with two differing levels of adjustment, dealing with their own reactions and those of others. One participant commented, 'All of the focus is on the victim, the focus is not on the family, and they've got to get through it. They are the ones who really need the help' (Plant, 1995, p.137).

The suffering of families indicated is also demonstrated by Wilson (1991) in her grounded theory study of husbands' experiences of their wives' chemotherapy. Although the husbands felt involved in the care process, they struggled constantly with suffering and endured this over long periods of time. Evidence of disease ramifications upon the family is apparent in a number of published studies that explore the needs of caregivers (Finch, 1996; Heileman, 1992; Lewis, 1993; Longman, 1992; Marcus-Lewis, 1998; Silveira and Winstead-Fry, 1997; Stetz *et al.*, 1996; Steele and Fitch, 1996). Most of this evidence originates in North America and is of limited generalisability of in a UK context; useful insights are, however, offered into the needs of different groups of patients. For example, in a qualitative study of bone marrow transplantation, five major themes arose from focus group interviews (Stetz *et al.*, 1996). The researcher set out to determine the information needs of families and demonstrated the theme of 'Preparing for caregiving', the seeking and acquisition of information related to diagnosis and treatment and an assessment of the validity of that information. Sub-themes of providing physical care, protecting, maintaining the patient's connection with life and advocating, were conceptualised as 'Managing the Care'. 'Facing Challenges' and 'Developing Supportive Strategies', all were part of the needs and experiences seen in this research group. Unexpectedly, family cohesion and personal growth were identified as a consequence of transplantation, with 'Discovering Unanticipated Rewards and Benefits' being the final theme to arise from the data. These findings suggest that family care-givers face challenges associated primarily with personal and interpersonal stress through the marrow transplant experience.

Family members of those undergoing cancer treatment demonstrate needs in relation to three distinct areas – personal care, involvement with healthcare and interpersonal interaction. Needs in relation to personal care includes a need to be assured their relative is comfortable, a need to know what symptoms to expect and how to observe effects of treatment. Needs related to involvement with healthcare, include a need for assurance of hospital re-admission if appropriate, emergency help, and need for information of their relatives condition and reports of changes in condition. Identified needs in relation to interpersonal interaction relate to communication with the patient and comfort and support needs from other family members (Longman *et al.*, 1992; Silveira and Winstead-Fry, 1997). Family care-givers of those receiving terminal care require information about the patient's condition and side effects of treatment (Hinds, 1985; Steele and Fitch, 1996; Duke *et al.*, 1998). In aspects such as patient care, for example, pain management, how to get patients to eat, ways to deal with patients' decreased energy and indicators of deterioration and death (Steele and Fitch, 1996); and household functions, for example community or voluntary services (Hinds, 1985). Care-givers demonstrate repeatedly a need for time to themselves (Hinds, 1985; Steele and Fitch, 1996; Duke *et al.*, 1998) and this is more evident in the families of terminally ill patients than in other groups (Heileman, 1992). Dealing with stress, and particularly guilt feelings, and information in relation to these psychological issues have been identified in at least two research groups (Hull, 1990; Steele and Fitch, 1996). In the majority of studies there is consistent evidence of unmet need, although the extent varies between studies.

The family needs assessment studies referred to above are all 'snapshot' surveys conducted at one specific period although they represent different examples within the cancer trajectory. A limited number of studies have utilised a longitudinal study design that has enabled evaluation of the impact of cancer on subject groups at various stages of the disease trajectory. For example, the work of Lewis, Hammond and Woods (1993); Issel, Esrek and Lewis (1990) and Woods & Lewis (1995), which describes the level of psychosocial functioning of school age children and adolescents whose mother had cancer, enables evaluation of its impact in the initial acute diagnostic phase and during long-term rehabilitation. The majority of studies of families' needs and experiences have focused upon one specific part of the cancer trajectory, for example, in the diagnostic phase, treatment phase or at the terminal point of illness. While this work is useful in identifying the particular needs and concerns of families at different points in the illness, there is a virtual absence of consideration of the needs of families of patients with a poor prognosis on diagnosis. Lung cancer and pancreatic cancer are just two examples of a disease process which is normally characterised by rapid physical deterioration and early death following diagnosis. The complexities of needs and the particular experiences of this group of family care-givers are largely unknown. Likewise, the needs and experiences of specific groups appear to have been marginalised in clinical research. For example, a proportionately large number of studies of families' needs and experiences of cancer have focused upon breast cancer and the spouse. Other diseases have not received such attention. Moreover, within this work the study of the impact of cancer using non-traditional forms of the family as study samples, for example lesbian partnerships, are absent from the literature. The implications for practice here are obvious in that neglected groups will not be treated in an informed way.

Psycho-Social Morbidity in Family Members: Findings From Studies of Individuals

Research within nursing and psychology further illuminates the ramifications of cancer by demonstrating psychological disturbance in the family. Overt psychological morbidity is sometimes a result of cancer in the patient and in individual family members. One early example of this can be seen in Baider and De Nour (1984) who followed spouses of women with breast cancer and documented higher levels of psychological distress over time and lower levels of adjustment than in diagnosed women. Similarly, Hoskins (1997) found a high level of psychological distress in spouses of women with breast cancer. In this descriptive survey Hoskins identified unmet interaction and emotional needs and the presence of negative emotions in spouses at various intervals up to one year following initial surgery. Negative emotions of gloom, tension, feelings of worry, being uneasy or troubled, decreased with time in the research population of 174 couples. This improvement in psychological well-being of both partners was related to successful surgery and recovery. Very soon following surgery husbands reported greater dissatisfaction with the extent to which patients agreed with their thinking, were open in communication of feelings and perceptions, or were sensitive or insightful of their feelings. Although this group showed improvement over time, it has been found that for some family members there is a significant decline in mental health (Ell *et al.*, 1988). Findings such as these take on greater significance in the light of current evidence and in consideration of trends in care and professional ideals for care of the dying. Current professional nursing discourses emphasise the home as an 'ideal place to die', if of course this is what the individual wishes. However, recent evidence suggests that informal carers of cancer patients, who die at home, fare less well than informal carers of those who die elsewhere. Bereaved respondents of deceased who died at home showed significantly higher levels of psychological distress and significantly worse adjustment to bereavement. The findings of Addington-Hall (1998) suggest that caring for a dying cancer patient at home in some way places informal carers at a disadvantage while they come to terms with their loss. The reasons why this may be so can only be hypothesised at this stage.

Psychosocial Morbidity: Findings From Studies of Family Units

The impact of cancer on the family and the impact of the family on illness have been examined earlier. While these two key notions are informed by differing theoretical perspectives and research traditions, namely social support and family nursing, they share one important element in their consideration of social relationships and family functioning, in that their analysis centres upon individual components which make up a greater whole. This notion is central to general systems theory (Bertalanffy, 1968), which informs many of the theoretical frameworks and explanations of family nursing. Systems theory views persons as more than the sum of individual parts, being complex, interrelated parts of a whole in continual interaction with each other. This theoretical assumption has been tested by the Family Functioning Research Team in the School of Nursing, University of Washington. Their family-level research relating to cancer has evolved from descriptive studies, to studies of relationships between subsets of family adjustment variables, to statistical modelling to test interrelated hypotheses.

The mediating effects of different variables have been identified by few nurse researchers in this field. Hoskins (1997) identified differences in adjustment between women with breast cancer and their spouses and raised further hypotheses in relation to some unexpected findings. At initial testing, and at each subsequent retest interval, husbands' and wives' perceptions of dissatisfaction, or satisfaction, with the extent to which a partner was meeting their needs were reversed, that is, diametrically opposed. Husbands therefore reported most dissatisfaction in relation to the extent to which their emotional and interaction needs were being met at 7–10 days, two months, and six months. Wives' patterns were reversed to their husbands in that they expressed most dissatisfaction at one month, three months and one year and in relation to interactional and emotional needs. This complex dynamic is explained by the researcher in the light of previous studies, for example the communication theory of Watzlawick (1967), which characterises such a relationship in terms of one partner occupying a relatively superior position and the other a corresponding secondary position. This pattern is explained as being prone to rigidity. The effects of cancer here accentuated the dynamics of a rigid pattern in interaction as a means of coping with the distressing experience. This study not only reveals evidence of suffering in a family member but shows there are differences in the concerns and needs of the spouse and patient and that these cannot be viewed in isolation from each other as they impact upon each other.

The notion of the family as an interdependent system is further illuminated in a longitudinal study of 80 mothers diagnosed with breast cancer, their male partners, school-aged children and adolescents (Lewis, 1998). A core set of processes of family adjustment to breast cancer were identified whereby greater illness demands caused an increase in parental depressed mood that, in turn, negatively affected the appraisal of their marriage. More illness related pressures caused increasingly negative views of marital quality. Families in which marriages were less well adjusted were also those that less frequently modified their coping behaviour in response to illness related pressures. The ability of the family to 'self-right' was hampered by marital tension. Self-monitoring, self-correcting and feedback-giving coping behaviour were identified as significant predictors of higher levels of successful functioning in the children and total household. Concepts of wholeness, feedback and homeostasis that are evidenced here are central tenets of general systems theory. Critical consideration of systems theory is essential to family nursing as many of the current ideas and beliefs supporting theory are built upon this approach. The remainder of this discussion will attempt to evaluate the usefulness of contemporary perspectives on therapeutic nursing within the family.

Where are the Boundaries of Family Nursing Practice in Cancer and Palliative Care?

Family Nursing Theory and Issues for Cancer and Palliative Care

In her study of families' experiences of cancer Plant (1995) noted that current philosophies of care include both family and patient. However, despite notions of 'family-centred care' an overwhelming feature of her interviews was the lack of contact families had with health professionals. Moreover, she acknowledged that in practice there is little time to investigate the intricacies of family networks. This view is opposed by many who see potential for nursing in this area to be not only effective but efficient, for example, by patients making fewer presentations to healthcare providers in the longer term. Although the concerns of patients and families living with cancer are complex, Altschul (1997) argued they should be central to nursing care and that nursing's thinking should increasingly replace the concept of the individual patient with that of the family.

Levels of Family Nursing

Family centred, or family focused care, are more frequently used terms within the UK which describe nurses' concerns with the patient's significant others. Family nursing is distinct from these concepts in that the family itself is seen as the unit of care, rather than the mere context for care. A distinction is made in the literature between generalist nurses who predominantly use the conceptualisations of family as context and specialists who work at the family systems level, viewing the family as the unit or client of care. The work of Friedman (1998) for defines different 'levels' of family nursing and her theory goes some way to defining the skills and competencies of 'general', 'specialist', and 'higher level practitioners', with regard to family care.

- Level one: The family is viewed insofar as it provides the context to client care.

- Level two: The family is seen as an accumulation or sum of its individual parts when care is available or provided for all family members.

- Level three: Nursing practice focuses upon family sub-systems with family dyads, triads and other sub-systems being the unit of analysis and care.

- Level four: The entire family is viewed as client and focus of assessment and care. Connections between illness, family members and the family are assessed and analysed. The nurse's role is to offer alternative perspectives to the problem, through the use of questions that introduce notions of circular versus linear relationships, patterns of interaction between persons, problems and environment and reciprocity.

The forms of nursing care described by Friedman most certainly represent a considerable advancement in practice for most nurses within the United Kingdom. However, like Whyte (1997), this generalisation needs to be qualified with apologies to those nurses who are already practising in this way.

Family Nursing or Family Therapy?

In analysing what constitutes the scope of nursing's practice with the family, the work of Whyte (1997) and Friedman (1998) shifts boundaries, at least in a theoretical sense with the blurring of professional boundaries between family nursing and family therapy. The orientation toward health is one major feature that Whyte sees as distinguishing family nursing from family therapy, whose traditional focus lies in family pathology. These definitions, however, fail to hold up to the scrutiny of contemporary theoretical approaches to family therapy in the context of postmodern society characterised by diversity, fragmentation plurality and a qualitatively expanded scope of social change. The challenges of 'postmodernity' are radical since they represent a crisis of a whole way of understanding the social world, or a fundamental change in the nature of social thought. Incredulity toward existing forms of knowledge defines the postmodern for Lyotard (1984). Ways in which these ideas are articulated within practice-based disciplinary ideas, are ably demonstrated by Brown & Christensen (1999). A key aspect of their theoretical model of family therapy is to 'normalise family struggles' or 'de-pathologise the family and the actions of its members'. Thus definitions of family therapy appear to be more similar than dissimilar to family nursing. However, multiple family therapy theories exist, the preponderance of which are concerned with the development of prescriptive practice-based interventions with 'dysfunctional families'. Structural Family Therapy Theory (Minuchin *et al.*, 1967), Experiential Humanistic Family Theory (Satir, 1972; Whitaker, 1976) and Behaviour Family Therapy Theory (Levant, 1980) are all examples of family therapy theories that cumulatively offer much in scientific understanding of families experiencing problems. As such they form part of the body of knowledge that must inform the work of the knowledgeable cancer or palliative care nurse wishing to develop in practice with families. Family therapy theories are one source of theoretical knowledge of the family, with social science theories, family nursing theories and clinical nursing research studies being other relevant sources.

Theoretical Foundations: Systems Theory and Family Development Theory

Systems theory and developmental theory, from the social sciences, appear to be fundamental to current scholarly nursing thought concerning family nursing. In this respect they share their origins with family systems therapy. Systems theory focuses upon relationship orientated events and on the interrelationships of parts to one another, rather than the parts that make up a whole (Bertalanffy, 1969). The process whereby all the family members operate together is referred to as the family system which relates to the community and the larger societal system and smaller systems of individuals. Family systems function by seeking stability and equilibrium or homeostasis. The individual units in the system communicate with each other through a process of circular feedback, with change in one area producing change in another (therefore communication and feedback mechanisms between family members are important in determining the behaviour of family members). The concept of wholeness arises from the interrelatedness of the system, whereby any effect will reverberate throughout the entire system (thus parts of the family are re-related to each other). This raises two key points; first, that the system cannot be scrutinised or understood through examination of the individual parts (one part of the family cannot be understood in isolation from the rest of the system), and second, that the effect of change in the system will impact upon all parts of the system (family functioning is therefore more than just a sum of its parts). The concept of boundaries is important as the integrity of each individual depends on a personal boundary while permeability allows for interaction and communication. A family's structure and organisation are important in determining the behaviour of family members to the extent which they represent a coherent or exclusive unit. Nurses may be permitted to move in and out of the family system if the family boundary is sufficiently permeable (Whyte, 1997). On the other hand they may not and the work of Plant (1995) suggests this may not necessarily be the case in families with a member newly diagnosed with cancer.

Family developmental theory provides a second example of social science family theory. This perspective focuses upon life cycle transitions and predictable, and unpredictable, developmental stressors and can be seen

Table 6.1   Family nursing assessment

Area assessed	Focus of Assessment
STRUCTURAL	
Family composition	Identification of key family members or informal support network. Level of support identified. Diagrammatically represented.
Family context	Culture, ethnicity, religion, social class, living environment, neighbourhood, financial resources.
DEVELOPMENTAL	Family's present developmental stage nuclear family history, life events, history of parents developmental tasks, attachments.
FUNCTIONAL	Activities of daily living, problem solving, health awareness family values, social support and boundaries communication, verbal and non-verbal roles, emotional involvement, coping strategies.

Note: Adapted from whyte (1997).

informing the work of family nursing theorists such as Dorothy Whyte at the University of Edinburgh. Other theoretical frameworks commonly seen in conceptualisations of family nursing include interactional theory (Hill and Hansen, 1960; Turner, 1970); stress theory (Artinian, 1994) and change theory (Maturana, 1978). Thus family nursing theories are models for nursing assessment and intervention that are grounded in the tradition of social sciences.

Nursing Assessment of the Family

A nursing assessment of family functioning devised by Whyte (1997) can be seen therefore to be composed of three qualitatively different sources of information:

1. structural: family composition and context;

2. developmental: present developmental stage of the family

3. functional: problem solving, health beliefs, emotional involvement and family coping, and social support boundaries (see Table 6.1).

Unfortunately the theory proposed by Whyte (1997) has not been applied to cancer or palliative care nursing, at least not as evidenced within the literature. This does not hold true for many of the other family nursing models, however, these are largely examples within American texts and they constitute, in the main, applied examples, rather than tested theories in research studies. One illustrative example of an assessment of family functioning in breast cancer can be seen in Bell's interview guide based on the Calgary Family Assessment Model (Wright and Leahy, 1994). Areas of assessment include beliefs and perceptions of cancer, emotional communication patterns in the family, and problem solving approaches.

As most family nursing theorists use a problem solving, or diagnostic, framework the assessment phase is followed by an intervention stage. A large number of specific nursing interventions are presented within the literature and may be of use to cancer or palliative care nurses extending the boundaries of practice with families. These strategies are in the main supported theoretically, rather than empirically, and also through case study work with feedback and reflection being offered by family members. Some of the interventions suggested by Wright and Leahy (1994) and Whyte (1997) are circular questioning, information and education, commending family and individual strengths, and reframing. Agreement of goals and tasks, empowerment strategies, lifestyle modification, including stress management, role modelling and social support and social network interventions are also deemed appropriate interventions within the family nursing literature (Friedman 1992, 1998; Stewart, 1993). The central philosophy underpinning the nursing approach is one of partnership, of working with families, helping them to identify concerns and mobilise their own coping resources, and in this is consistent with the philosophies of cancer and palliative care nursing. The extent to which individual interventions are useful and acceptable to families with a member with cancer or terminal illness, is largely unknown.

Case Example

Assessment

Ms C, aged 53, has advanced pancreatic cancer with liver metastases. Post-surgery she developed a deep vein thrombosis, and has gross swelling of her left leg that renders her virtually immobile. Her general condition can best be described as poor and debilitated, she has intractable nausea despite the palliative care team's best efforts at symptom control. She has eaten little for the past month and has experienced considerable weight loss. She has hospital acquired Multi-resistant staphylococcus-aureus (MRSA) following surgery.

Structural Family Composition and Context

Ms C is the main carer for her 95-year-old mother. They have lived together always. Ms C has two sisters and four nephews who offer a high level of practical support, including attending to her physical needs, for example washing, providing comfort, cooking and housework. Each family member takes it in turns to spend the night. They live in a working-class neighbourhood on an estate that has become more troubled and deprived in recent years. There is a large drug problem in the area. The financial resources of Ms C and her mother are just about adequate for their needs.

Developmental Assessment

Ms C has never married. She has no intimate personal relationship at present. Ms C has a close relationship with her sisters; they are both considerably older than she is as she was a late younger child in the family. Nearing their seventies, their general health is not good. Ms C's mother is very dependent on her, emotionally rather than physically. Since the death of her father 30 years ago they have lived together, alone. Other members of the family observe that their relationship is one of co-dependency. Mrs C is the 95-year-old matriarch in the family, the others pay her respect and defer to her, as they have done for all of their lives. Ms C has a long and close connection with her church and has numerous friends from the congregation.

Functional Assessment

Ms C is still struggling to accept her diagnosis and deteriorating state of health. She is very frightened and will often wake during the night in terror. The family is able to communicate openly about Ms C's fears of her impending death, but they find this very painful. Ms C's nausea is fairly constant, most of her energies when awake are spent trying to manage and cope with this experience.

Ms C's mother has difficulty sleeping, she sometimes becomes confused at night and will wander the house waking Ms C and a family carer. It is not unusual for Mrs C to get fully dressed three or more times during the night. She then needs help to get undressed and return to bed.

Ms C was not expecting a diagnosis of cancer; it was discovered during investigation for a more 'routine' health problem. She was initially optimistic about the future but this did not last long as her physical condition deteriorated rapidly. It is four months since diagnosis.

Mrs C's mother is very angry with her for being ill, as she is no longer able to care for her needs adequately.

Crisis/Problem for the family

The individual members of the family are in conflict and disagreement arising from an aspect of Ms C's management. Her prothrombin time is erratic and she has been asked to return to the hospital three times a week to have this monitored by the surgical team, at the request of the surgeon. The journey to the hospital is traumatic for all of those involved. Ms C is in intense pain when travelling the distance by car and when moving from car to clinic. She vomits during the journey. She has a long wait to be seen by the medical staff and is disappointed that instead of seeing the surgeon she sees a different junior doctor on each occasion. Because of her MRSA she needs to shower prior to the hospital visit. The visit leaves her exhausted and dispirited.

Some family members are incensed with this aspect of Ms C's management and they wish to ask the GP to find alternative arrangements. Ms C does not wish to 'cause trouble', it is her view that the surgical team are monitoring her health and 'so be it'. Everyone in 'the family' appears tired and distressed. They are in disagreement about what, if any, action is to be taken.

Summary of Nursing Intervention

Assessment indicated that problem solving in the family was disrupted, even blocked. Open communication and feedback from nurse to family members offered alternative interpretations of others' perspectives. Wright and Leahy (1994) state that the nurse's role is to offer new perspectives to the problem. The use of circular questions promotes reflection and open possibilities for change. Future orientated in nature they enable families to focus on the future rather than the present. Families coping with serious health problems find it difficult to focus on the future because they are so preoccupied with present difficulties and so fearful of the future. This attitude inhibits problem-solving attempts. Questions such as 'What are you worried will happen if you ask your GP to reconsider your care?' revealed fears of abandonment from the healthcare team. 'If things continue going the way they are now, what do you will expect will become of the family in the medium term' facilitated reflection and a desire to change the situation in relation to the hospital visit and support for carers at night.

In the experience of Wright and Leahy (1994) and in this example, interventive questions have been sufficient to effect change within families that have difficulty dealing with their crisis.

Challenges for Family Nursing

The scholarly contributions of Whyte (1997) and Friedman (1998) are significant as they provide a challenge for nursing in relation to its scope of practice with the family. However, as global, overarching and eclectic theories, which sometimes incorporate a number of mid range theories, they are useful in describing a family approach but less useful in offering prescriptive or intervention strategies. The approach of family nursing espoused by Whyte (1997), Friedman (1998) and (Wright and Leahy, 1994) will remain undetermined by evidence because of the global and eclectic nature of the theory. So while current family nursing theories offer much in terms of a philosophy of nursing they appear to have less to offer in terms of testable practice outcomes. This is regrettable as very many important research questions remain. For example, are family nursing interventions acceptable to the population of people with cancer and their families and are they effective in improving health? Are they acceptable to specialist and higher level nursing practitioners in cancer and palliative care, and in which context, the acute care environment, community or palliative setting? Questions must be asked concerning the effectiveness of models of family focused services particularly in an environment of cost constraints. Perhaps as service models those practitioners offering family focused care could be compared with those who offer individualised care, the predominant model of service delivery in current practice. Lastly, but not of least importance, the education and training needs of nurses advancing their practice in family nursing must be established.

Family nursing offers a new way to look at practice and it raises many challenges. For example new ethical dilemmas may be faced in relation to confidentiality and autonomy, where patients needs conflict with the needs of others in the family. Issues such as safe practice must be addressed as the interventions and approaches defined within the literature have potentially harmful as well as therapeutic effects. While Keeling *et al.* (1996) acknowledge the potential untherapeutic and practical problems of working at a group level, others such as family nursing theorists, largely ignore this issue. While the scope of practice remains within the domain of health promotion with the family, rather than dealing with family problems, these issues must be addressed in education and training and supervision and support. The specific educational and training needs of cancer and palliative care practitioners in relation to family care are largely unknown.

While the Post-Registration and Practice Project (PREP) (UKCC, 1994) of specialist community nursing practice identifies learning outcomes related to the care of families other nurses' contributions are not identified. However, Whyte (1997) believes that those in specialist or advanced roles in practice will look for help in developing their role to meet clients needs more effectively and in so doing will provide nurse education with a challenge. The skills and qualities required of the family nurse are not those expected in primary practice, Whyte argues, but are those attributes inherent in higher level, or advanced practice. And thus the nurse practising family nursing inherently displays; independent decision making and sophisticated use of clinical knowledge, systematic assessment and intervention, high levels of accountability and expansion of the boundaries of nursing practice (Read and Graves, 1994).

Development of these complex interpersonal elements of the nursing role must be accompanied by high quality relevant education and training and skilled clinical supervision. Moreover the vision for developments in family nursing practice in cancer and palliative care will only be sustained if the benefits are clearly articulated in positive patient and family outcomes. Systematic evaluation and research of family nursing interventions is therefore imperative.

Evaluating the Evidence Base for a Family Nursing Approach in Cancer and Palliative Care

To date, only a handful of scientists and clinicians have developed and scientifically evaluated family-focused interventions for families affected by cancer (Samarel, Fawcett and Tulman, 1992; Telch and Telch, 1986; Lewis, 1998). An example of a superior study, demonstrating excellence in cancer nursing research, can be seen in a clinical trial intervention for families with children whose mothers were diagnosed with breast cancer (Lewis, 1998). Over a 15-year period, the family functioning research team at the School of Nursing, University of Washington, have undertaken empirical research within several phases. The first phase research involved clinical practice papers that heightened awareness about the potential negative impact of cancer upon the individual and family. The second phase relied primarily on cross-sectional research designs using standardised measures of psychosocial functioning which involved descriptions of the level, intensity, frequency and domains of psychosocial morbidity. Longitudinal data revealed important data, for example that spouse's distress increased not decreased over time (Baider and De-Nour, 1984). Relationships between subsets of family variables, such as social support and marital quality were examined in these studies (Primoro *et al.*,

1990; Yates *et al.*, 1995). The third phase of the studies went further to include the use of statistical modelling techniques to test interrelated hypotheses about the impact of breast cancer on the family (Lewis and Hammond, 1992, 1996; Woods and Lewis, 1995). This work attempted to model the complexity of family life. Family system intervention studies used the knowledge generated in the three phases described. Results from previous studies revealed that family members were affected by the woman's breast cancer in four ways: by direct impact from the illness related pressures, by direct impact from either parent's direct mood, by tension in the marriage related to the illness and by the relative absence of coping resources to existing illness related pressures. Specifically, in studies of those experiencing a recent or long term diagnosis, marital quality significantly predicted the level of the family's adjustment in an array of family system variables, including the quality of parenting, the frequency with which families coped with problems and their cohesion and adaptability. Based on these results a multi-component intervention, The Family Home Visitation Program, was developed for use with couples.

The family program components consisted of an integration of an emotive-expressive, cognitive behavioural, and competency based management model of adjustment to illness (Meyerowitz *et al.*, 1983; Telch and Telch, 1986; Lewis and Daltroy, 1990). The specific goals of the intervention being to increase the woman's and husband's cognitive-behavioural control over managing the impact of cancer in their family member's daily lives, minimise their depressed mood, decrease the number of illness related demands experienced and increase the quality of their dyadic relationship. The standard, protocol driven intervention had three components. Firstly couples were invited to discuss their concerns, and areas of difficulty (their 'stuck points') with cancer. This was followed by work with the couples to augment their knowledge, skills and cognitive behavioural control. Most aspects of the intervention were identified by previous research, with Social Cognitive Theory informing the mechanism whereby control could be enhanced. However, another component was added to the intervention to enhance self care and self-efficacy in the couple. This involved the operationalisation of the construct of 'nurse as coach'. The couple was thus experts, learners and self-care agents with the nurse as facilitator/enhancer (Benner, 1984, 1985; Benner and Wrubel, 1989; Lewis and Zahilis, 1997).

The nurse as coach was demonstrated in six dimensions:

- attending to the story
- encircling the experience
- inviting the work (taking a piece of it and making the work safe)

- exploring solutions (advocating further movement and learning from the past)
- anchoring the skill
- setting up success.

Subsequently participants in this randomised, longitudinal study demonstrated significant changes for women on the assessment of the quality of their marriage when compared with controls. No significant differences existed between intervention and control group on any other outcomes, including cognitive behavioural control, illness related demands and depressed mood. In contrast intervention husbands benefited in three areas – cognitive behavioural control, depressed mood and marital adjustment, with illness-related demands not changing. Clearly there is still much to be achieved in research aimed at helping couples when the woman has breast cancer.

Accumulated evidence from findings in the family functioning research team suggests that families do not always function in ways predicted in the literature. Over time (Lewis, 1998), suggests that families stabilise or 'freeze' in the ways they function as a household. They do not appear to operate as dynamic systems that modify what they do as a function of the illness specific issues they are exposed to. The finding that family functioning is more responsive to tension in the marriage than illness-related demands, leads Lewis to conclude that the family is managing its core functions as a family, rather than it is managing the illness-related pressures, put upon it by the mother's cancer. She therefore concludes that the mother's cancer is 'put under the table, not on top of it'. She goes on to question the appropriateness of the use of a cognitive-behavioural model of intervention in the early stages of illness as this may not be a 'best fit' when illness-related demands are dominant issues for the couple. Thus different models of intervention, derived from different theoretical perspectives, deserve attention and evaluation in different stages of cancer. Significant advances in practice, in cancer and palliative care, must therefore be accompanied by the development of new knowledge of family functioning and its response to specialist and advanced nursing care.

The development of new knowledge in care of the family with a life threatening illness causes many challenges to researchers. Major conceptual and methodological issues facing family researchers include, defining the family, determining the unit of analysis in the level of inquiry and research design. Defining the family is an important concern since the definition has implications for sampling and measurement (Feetham, 1991; Kristjanson, 1986). However, McClement and Woodgate (1997) argue that most definitions tend to be too stringent or too vague. Definitions which are 'exclusive' and do not account for today's multiple family forms; for example, single parents, same sex couples, are of course problematic in contemporary pluralist society. Concept analysis of the 'family' fails to clarify differences between an ad hoc small group or social support network (Stuart, 1991). The family unit as identified by the patient as 'being important' may be the best definition for research and practical purposes, however, there must be a recognition that this 'family member-ship' can change over the course of an illness. Researchers must not only decide how the family will be defined, but also decide which members will be the unit of analysis. So while some researchers focus upon individual members others, who use a systems framework, see the whole family as the unit of analysis. Further methodological challenges in cancer and palliative care include, in qualitative research, problems of eliciting in-depth data from a variety of informants with Casseleth *et al.* (1985) noting participation in research 'may be impossible for one, let alone multiple family members experiencing high levels of anxiety and emotional distress'. In quantitative research, with the notable exceptions of Kristjanson (1986) and Lewis (1998) there are relatively few tools developed with popu-lations of palliative and cancer patients. There are clearly real challenges to be faced in order to advance knowledge in this area. Despite these, and other difficulties not referred to in this brief paper, there is a need for high quality outcome based studies of nursing practice with the family.

Discussion

In their daily, experiences of nursing patients with a terminal illness, or with cancer, nurses witness the distress and suffering of family members. In the majority of healthcare encounters nurses demonstrate support and empathy toward the family and include them in care and decisions regarding care, when the patient deems this appropriate. Most, however, operate at the level of viewing the family as context. Few systematically work with the family unit as described in the earlier discussion. The reality is that nurses care about families, but caring about the family is different from servicing the family in a structured way. Both Friedman (1998) and Lewis (1998), while acknowledging developments in theory and research, lament the contrast between what is promulgated and what is practised. While there are certain minima that must occur when patients are put on a new chemotherapy protocol, no such rules exist for interventions that aim to diminish the impact of cancer on the everyday life and relationships of the family. Models of care focused upon family services could, and prob-ably should, consist of minimum, intermediate and case intensive standards (Lewis, 1998). Certainly it is apparent that practice development in this area must be accompanied by service development and generation of new knowledge of family functioning. However, it may be that family nursing is just 'wishful thinking'; a nice idea, certainly in theory, but not appropriate or feasible in the daily practice of cancer and palliative care nurses. If nurses are to push back boundaries and advance their care in response to patient need so clearly evidenced within the literature, they need to lobby for improvement in services, influence decision makers, pilot and test innovative and efficient methods of care delivery, (perhaps making greater use of information technology), raise research questions, and participate in the evaluation of research as it is relevant and appropriate for their practice. Clearly much is to be achieved if nursing is to demonstrate health and healing with families in this context.

References

Addington-Hall, J.M (1998) Do informal carers of cancer patients who die at home fare less well in bereavement than informal carers of patients who die elsewhere? *Annual Palliative Care Congress*, 15–17 September, University of Leeds.

Altschul, A. (1997) Foreword, in D.A. Whyte (Ed.), *Explorations in Family Nursing*. London: Routledge.

Artinian, N.T. (1994) Selecting a model to guide family assessment. *Dimensions of Critical Care Nursing*, 14(1), 4–16.

Baider, L. and A.K. De Nour (1984) Couples' reactions and adjustment to mastectomy: A preliminary report. *International Journal of Psychiatry in Medicine*, 14, 265–75.

Benner, P. (1984) *From Novice to Expert*. Menlo Park, CA: Addison-Wesley.

Benner, P. (1985) The oncology clinical specialist: an expert coach, *Oncology Nursing Forum*, 12(2), 40–44.

Benner, P. and J. Wrubel (1989) *The Primacy of Caring*. Menlo Park, CA: Addison-Wesley.

Bertalanffy, L. von (1968) *General Systems Theory*. New York: Braziller.

Bowlby, J. (1969) *Attachment and Loss*, Vol. 1. New York: Basic Books.

Brown, J. and D. Christensen (1999) *Family Therapy Theory and Practice*. 2nd edn. London: Brooks/Cole.

Carlsson, M. and E. Hamrin (1994) Psychological and psychosocial aspects of breast cancer and breast cancer treatment: a literature review. *Cancer Nursing*, 7(5), 418–28.

Cassileth B.R., E.J. Lusk and T.B. Strouse (1985) A psychological analysis of cancer patients and their next of kin. *Cancer*, 5, 72–6.

Cobb, S. (1976) Social support as a moderator of life stress. *Psychosomatic Medicine*, 38(5), 300–14.

Costain-Schou, K. and J. Hewison (1999) *Experiencing Cancer*. Buckingham: Open University Press.

Coyne, J.C., C. Wortman and D.R. Lehman (1998) The other side of support: emotional over involvment and miscarried help, in B.H. Gottileb (ed.), *Marshalling Social Support*, Newbury Park, CA: Sage, pp. 305–30.

Dakof, G. and S. Taylor (1990) Victim's perceptions of social support: what is helpful and from whom?, *Journal of Personality and Social Psychology*, 58(1), 80–89.

Duke, S., S. Prowse, J. Fancott and J. Dancer (1998) An assessment of palliative care needs as perceived by people with progressive illness, their family carers and healthcare professionals. *Annual Palliative Care Congress*, 15–17 September, University of Leeds.

Dunkel-Schetter, C. (1984) Social support and cancer: findings based on patent interviews and their implications. *Journal of Social Issues*, 40(4), 77–98.

Dunkel-Schetter, C., D. Blasband, L. Feinstein and T. Bennett (1992) Elements of supportive interactions: When are attempts to help effective?, in S. Spacapan and S. Oskamp (eds), *Helping and Being Helped in the Real World*. Newbury Park, CA: Sage.

Durkheim, E. (1981) *Suicide: A study in sociology.* J.A. Spalding and Thompson translation. New York: Academic Press.

Ell, K., R. Nishimoto, J. Mantell and M. Hamovitch (1988) Longitudinal analysis of psychological adaptation among family members of patients with cancer. *Journal of Psychosomatic Research,* 32(4/5), 429–38.

Fallowfield, L. 1990 Psychosocial adjustment after early treatment for breast cancer. *Oncology* 4(4), 89–97.

Feetham, S.L. (1991) Conceptual and methodological issues in search of families, in E. Whall and J. Fawcett (eds), *Family Theory Development in Nursing: State of the Science and Art.* Massachusetts: F.A. Davis.

Finch, J. (1996) Family Responsibilities and Rights, in M. Bulmer and A.M. Rees (eds), *Citizenship Today: the contemporary relevance of T.H. Marshall.* London: UCL Press, pp. 193–8.

Friedman, M. (1992) *Family Nursing: Research, Theory and Practice.* 2nd edn. Connecticut: Appleton & Lange.

Friedman, M. (1998) *Family Nursing: Research, Theory and Practice.* 4th edn. Stamford, CT: Appleton & Lange.

Heileman, J. (1992) Identifying the needs of home care givers of patients with cancer. *Oncology Nursing Forum,* 19, 771–7.

Hill, R. and D. Hansen (1960) The identification of a conceptual framework utilised in a family study. *Marriage and Family Nursing,* 22(4), 299–311.

Hinds, C. (1985) What are the needs of the terminally ill dying at home? *Journal of Advanced Nursing,* 10, 230–38.

Hoskins, C.N. (1997) Differences in adjustment between women with breast cancer and their spouses: implications for nursing interventions. *Clinical Effectiveness in Nursing,* 1, 105–11.

Hull, M. (1990) Sources of stress for hospice caregiving families. *The Hospice Journal,* 6(2), 29–53.

Issel, L.J., M. Eresk and F.M. Lewis (1990) How children cope with mother's breast cancer. *Oncology Nursing Forum,* 17, 5–13.

Keeling, D.I., P.E. Price, E. Jones and K.G. Harding (1996) Social support: some pragmatic implications for health care professionals. *Journal of Advanced Nursing,* 23(1): 76–81.

Krishnasamy, M. (1996) Social support and the patient with cancer: a review of the literature. *Journal of Advanced Nursing,* 23(4), 757–62.

Kristjanson, L.J. (1986) Indicators of quality of palliative care from a family perspective. *Journal of Palliative Care,* 2, 7–19.

Levant, R.F. (1980) Sociological and Clinical Models of the Family: An attempt to identify paradigms. *American Journal of Family Therapy,* 8, 5–20.

Lewis, F.M. (1993) Psychosocial transitions and the families work in adjusting to cancer. *Seminars in Oncology Nursing,* 9, 127–9.

Lewis, F.M. (1998) Family level services in oncology nursing: facts, fallacies, and realities revisited. *Oncology Nursing Forum,* 25(8), 1378–86.

Lewis, F.M. and L. Daltroy (1990) How Causal Explanations Influence Health Behavior: Attribution Theory, in K. Glanz, F.M. Lewis and B. Rimer (eds), *Health Behavior and Health Education: Theory, Research and Practice.* San Francisco: Jossey-Bass.

Lewis, F.M. and M.A. Hammond (1992) Psychological adjustment of the family to breast cancer: a longitudinal analysis. *Journal of the American Women's Association,* 47(5), 194–200.

Lewis, F.M., M.A. Hammond and N.F. Woods (1993) The Family's Functioning With Newly Diagnosed Breast Cancer in the Mother: the development of an exploratory model. *Journal of Behavioral Medicine,* 16(4), 351–70.

Lewis, F.M. and E.H. Zahilis (1997) The nurse as coach a conceptual framework for clinical practice. *Oncology Nursing Forum,* 26(8), 1695–1702.

Longman, A. (1992) Care needs of home based cancer patients and their caregivers. *Cancer Nursing,* 15, 182–90.

Longman, A.J., J.R. Atwood, J. Sherman, J. Benedict and C. Tsu-Ching Shang (1992) Care Needs of Home-based Cancer Patients and Their Care Givers. *Cancer Nursing,* 15(3), 182–90.

Lyotard, J.F. (1984) *The Post-modern Condition: A Report on Knowledge.* Manchester: Manchester University Press.

Marcus-Lewis, F. (1998) Family level services in oncology nursing: facts fallacies and realities re-visited. *Oncology Nursing Forum*, 25, 1378–87.

Maturana, H.R. (1978) Biology of language: the epistemology of reality, in G. Millar and E. Lenneberg (eds), *Psychology and biology of language and thought*. New York: Academic Press.

McClement, S.E. and R.L. Woodgate (1998) Research with families in palliative care: conceptual and methodological challenges. *European Journal of Cancer Care*, 7, 247–54.

Minuchin, S., B. Montalvo, B.G. Guerney, B.L. Rosman and F. Schumer. (1967) *Pyschosomatic Families*. Cambridge, MA: Harvard University Press.

Peters-Golden, H. (1982) Breast cancer: varied perceptions of social support in the illness experience. *Social Science and Medicine*, 16(4), 483–91.

Picardie, R. (1998) *Before I Say Goodbye*. London: Penguin.

Plant, H. (1995) The experiences of families of newly diagnosed cancer patients – selected findings, in A. Richardson and J. Wilson-Barnet (eds), *Nursing Research in Cancer Care*. London: Scutari Press.

Primomo, J., B.C. Yates and N.F. Woods (1990) Social Support and for women during chronic illness: the relationship among sources and types to adjustment. *Research in Nursing and Health*, 13(3), 153–61.

Read, S. and K. Graves (1994) Reduction of junior doctors hours' in Trent Region: The nursing contribution, in B. West (ed.), *Health service developments and the scope of professional nursing practice: a review of the pertinent literature*. Edinburgh: S.O.H.H.D.

Satir, V. (1972) *Peoplemaking*. London: Souvenir Press.

Silveira, J., and P. Winstead-Fry (1997) The Needs of Patients with Cancer and Their Carers in Rural Areas. *Oncology Nursing Forum*, 24(1), 71–6.

Steele, R. and M. Fitch (1996) Needs of family caregivers receiving home hospice care for cancer. *Oncology Nursing Forum*, 23(5), 823–8.

Stetz, K., J. McDonald and K. Compton (1996) Needs and experiences of family caregivers during marrow transplantation. *Oncology Nursing Forum*, 23(9), 1423–7.

Stewart, M.J (1993) *Integrating social support and nursing*. Newbury Park: Sage.

Stuart, M.E (1991) An analysis of the concept of family, in A.L. Whall and J. Fawcett (eds), *Family Theory Development in Nursing: State of the Science and Art*. Massachusetts: F.A. Davis.

Telch, C.F. and M.J. Telch (1986) Group coping skills instruction and supportive group therapy for cancer patients: A comparison of strategies. *Journal of Consulting and Clinical Psychology*, 54, 802–8.

UKCC (1994) *The Future of Professional Practice. The Council's Standards for Education and Practice Following Registration*. London: UKCC.

Turner, R.H. (1970) *Family Interaction*. New York: Wiley.

Watzlawick, P., J. Helmcik-Beavon and D.D. Jackson (1967) *Pragmatics of Human Communication: a study of interactional patterns, pathologies, and paradoxes*. New York: W.W. Norton.

Whyte, D. (1997) *Explorations in Family Nursing*. London: Routledge.

Whyte, D. and Y. Robb (1999) Families under stress how can nurses help? *Nursing Times*, 95(30), 50–51.

Wills, T.A. (1985) Supportive functions of interpersonal relationships in S. Cohen and L. Syme (eds), *Social Support and Health*. New York: Academic Press.

Wilson, S. (1991) The unrelenting nightmare: husbands experiences during their wives chemotherapy, in J. Morse (ed.), *The Illness Experience, Dimensions of Suffering*. London: Sage.

Woods, N.F. and F.M. Lewis (1995) Women with chronic illness: their views of their families' adaptation. *Health Care for Women International*, 16(2), 135–48.

Wortman, C. (1984) The Role of Social support in adaptation and recovery in physical illness, in C. Wortman and T. Conway (eds), *Social Support and Health*. New York: Academic Press.

Wright, L. and M. Leahy (1994) *Nurses and Families: A Guide to Family Assessment and Intervention*. 2nd edn. Philadelphia: F.A. Davis.

Yates, B.C., L.S. Bensley, B. Lalonde, F.M. Lewis, and N.F. Woods, (1995) The impact of marital status and quality of family functioning in maternal chronic illness. *Health Care for Women International*, 16(5), 437–49.

7

Spirituality: its Dynamics and Purpose in Nursing a Person With a New Diagnosis of Cancer

KEVIN KENDRICK and NIC HUGHES

At its most fundamental, a diagnosis of cancer threatens human life – unchallenged it will lead to death of the organism. Beyond this threat to the physical domain there is a commensurate violation of those borders that help an individual experience constancy, buoyancy and security. This is because, despite notable advances in treatments, therapies and survival rates, the popular psyche still views a diagnosis of cancer as a prelude to dying and death. Given this notoriety, there is little surprise that a diagnosis of cancer shakes individuals to the heart of their existential core (Weisman and Worden, 1976). This most fundamental human response is mirrored in classical and contemporary literature that describes death and dying in various ways: the end of an organism (Jasper, 1932), obscene, unmentionable, pornography – a nasty mistake (May, 1969), a crisis (Abiven, 1995), a period of suffering (Salt, 1997).

In this chapter, we offer a narrative that argues a person experiencing the trauma of a cancer diagnosis mirrors those features found in the concept of spiritual distress. In nursing, the language of spirituality is usually couched in terms that are synonymous with religion. This is vividly illustrated in nursing documents when information about a patient's religious faith is placed under the theme of spirituality; such thinking fails to address intrinsic differences between the two concepts. While religion may inform and offer direction to a person's spirituality, each has very different defining features. In terms of analogy, hydrogen and oxygen combine to make water but each brings its own essence to balance the chemical equation. For the most of the last century, researchers who explored the negative effects of religion often focused on specific beliefs and practices. More recently, studies examining the benefits of spirituality cite its role in personality integration, and a sense of harmony and meaning in life (Smucker, 1996). What emerges from this is that there may be a connection between religion and spirituality but that each has unique qualities that define their nature and purpose. Given this, a person's spirituality can thrive irrespective of a religious creed (Kendrick and Robinson, 2000).

Given that nursing has given spirituality a focus in the schema of care that is offered to patients, it places an obligation on nurses to be conversant with the concept and able to translate its themes to the processes associated with care delivery. If we cannot articulate what we mean by spirituality in the context of the nurse–patient relationship then its usefulness for our professional focus becomes questionable; quite simply, how can nurses offer spiritual care to patients with a diagnosis of cancer if they cannot articulate its defining characteristics? This lack of conceptual accuracy needs urgent clarification if this aspect of practice is to be advanced with regard to the care that nurses offer to people who are told they have a malignancy.

Spirituality Defined as a Search for Meaning and Purpose

Some commentators, for example Ross (1995), Oldnall (1996) and Long (1997) approach spirituality in terms of that which is concerned with a person's search for meaning and purpose. When spirituality is seen in this way it creates esoteric images that place the concept in the realm of the contemplative, enigmatic, abstract and mystical, rather than being seen as something that is intrinsically woven into the everyday themes and concerns of being human. Sitting, for example, on a hill thinking about the nature and purpose of being could certainly be seen as a spiritual exercise and may even form a spiritual experience. It does not, however, constitute the entire essence of spirituality but merely serves to show how some people may wish to engage in spiritual expression (Kendrick and Robinson, 2000).

When a person thinks about the meaning and purpose of a cancer diagnosis it is because the experience has imposed a captive state that moves the subjective gaze to the ontological. In essence, a person faced with an initial diagnosis of cancer is violated by an invading pathology that cannot be quelled by any measure of self or inner resource. No matter how sensitively such 'bad news' is revealed it confronts an individual's sense of being and casts it into turmoil and chaos. There is no chance or choice of looking away from the malignancy's presence; its terrifying occupancy haunts the lived experience as vividly as the lion that prowls the stricken antelope. Such themes are eloquently captured in the following piece from the journalist John Diamond mirroring his own reflections on being given a diagnosis of cancer:

> My cancer was, said Mr Mady [Diamond's doctor] on the phone that night, a squamous cell carcinoma, an indolent cancer, a cancer which – as if this would sugar the pill – surprised him as much as it did me. Not knowing about the 57 varieties, all I heard was that I had cancer. Mady didn't mention the natural corollary that I was going to die soon – but I supplied that for myself. For the one thing everyone knows about cancer is that it kills. There is no curing the cancer patient: the most that can be hoped for is a temporary remission while the appeal court argues about the precise date of execution (Diamond, 1998, p.37).

John Diamond's reflections about his own diagnosis of cancer are, in every way, very different from the person who sits on the hill thinking about purpose and meaning from the liberated state that health can afford and highlights the limitations of viewing spirituality in such a parochial way. What unites both situations, however, is that they can be seen as expressions of spirituality.

What has been emphasised here is that individuals with a new diagnosis of cancer are forced to confront existential concerns that focus upon the meaning of life, illness and possible death (O'Connor *et al.*, 1990). In essence, this search for meaning is a striving to understand and make order of the chaos that, so often, is intrinsic to receiving a diagnosis of malignancy. The importance of such themes is that illness and suffering cannot be brought into focus without taking into account personal meaning (Cassell, 1982). This search for meaning has been consistently coupled with spirituality (Frankl, 1978). The relevance of such elements for the professional gaze of the nurse has been described in the following way:

> The professional nurse hoping to deal with human responses in the fullest sense of the word 'human' must be prepared to assist individuals and families not just in coping with illness and suffering, but in finding meaning in these experiences (O'Connor *et al.*, 1990, p.168).

What has emerged so far is that the search for meaning and purpose, as evidenced by the literature, can be seen as a characteristic that helps to define the concept of spirituality. A more detailed narrative must be offered, however, if the fuller conceptual essence of spirituality is to be discerned in the relationship between nurse and the patient with a new diagnosis of cancer. This notion finds its ultimate convergence in the description of spirituality as a transcendent quality in human interaction that is more than a search for meaning and purpose; we return to this point later in the chapter.

Spirituality: the Whole of the Human Condition

Some writers, for example McSherry and Draper (1997), Engebretson (1996) and Emblem and Halstead (1993) have chosen to describe spirituality as a 'dimension' of the human situation. Such thinking evokes questions about the loci of spirituality and its relationship with other human domains, namely the somatic, psychical and social elements. When the term 'dimension' is used it suggests a concept of spirituality as something akin to an ethereal addendum that is loosely but indefinably connected to the human condition.

Semantics of this kind clearly suggest that spirituality is just part, rather than the whole, of the human condition. Here we are challenging such themes in favour of a language that presents spirituality as an orientation that is inclusive of all those elements that constitute the state of being human. Taking this further, there is no separate spiritual 'part' of the personality. Here we are using the term 'personality' in the classical sense to mean 'the dynamic organisation within the individual of those psychological systems that determine his or her unique adjustments to the environment' (Allport, 1937, p.48).

Spirituality is concerned with the whole personality and in particular with the development of awareness of the 'other' (for example, self, other person, wider communities, environment, deity). This evolving awareness is a dynamic process that involves a deepening integration of cognitive, affective, somatic and experiential knowledge. Spirituality thus seeks to make connections within the self and beyond the self; this finds strength and focus in the notions of integrity and shalom (peace with justice). Such themes offer some grounding on which individuals can base their *raison d'être* and a search for meaning. What emerges from this is that spirituality is an inclusive notion that captures every aspect of the human condition. To this end, we celebrate the sentiments expressed by Mayer (1992, p.55), 'If spirituality is seen as embracing the whole of what it is to be human, then the essence of spiritual care is not doctrine or dogma but the fundamental capacity to enter into the world of others and respond with feeling'.

Within this context, spirituality is what gives focus to the sum of all the parts that form the human condition and therefore, because of this entirety, cannot be reduced to the status of a single dimensional quality. Spirituality is not reliant upon religious, secular or agnostic themes but forms the very essence of the human person irrespective of which ideology that individual chooses to embrace. Oldnall (1996, p.144) has offered critical comment on this notion by arguing that:

> Spirituality is broader than the confines imposed from a purely religious or human-istic perspective, since the perceived spirit within each individual may be con-sidered as the driving force that gives meaning to life for that individual and in so doing helps to create a set of values and beliefs that can influence the conduct of their lives.

Oldnall's comments add vibrancy because they offer an interpretation of spirituality that goes beyond a search for meaning and purpose. This is evidenced by the dynamic notion that spirituality can inform a personal ethic and is translated to the influence of individual behaviour. What emerges from this is that spirituality has a transcendent quality oriented beyond the confines of the individual towards the focus of other concerns. This illustrates a relationship between the intra-personal, interpersonal and transpersonal. Yet a diagnosis of cancer, as we have already discussed, causes such existential plight that the usual sense of ecology between these three elements is utterly disrupted. In essence, this sense of angst, turmoil and chaos seems out of keeping with modern interpretations of spirituality that emphasis its role in personality integration, and a sense of harmony and meaning in life. Yet if, as we have argued here, spirituality is an inclusive concept that involves all of the human condition then a narra-tive must be offered that engages with a suitable vocabulary that describes spirituality in terms that are resonant with the lived experience of being told you have a malignancy.

Spiritual distress and the cancer diagnosis

Some commentators, for example Kaye and Robinson (1995), Granstrom (1985) and Baines (1984), have attempted to give examples of those human behaviours that typify the expression of spirituality. Taking this further, Kaye and Robinson (1995, p.220) have identified what they term 'spiritual behaviours' displayed by women whose partners have dementia; some of these behaviours were

- talking to friends or family about issues of concern
- interaction with a deity conceived as omniscient
- sharing the joys of living
- being able to embrace the essence of forgiveness.

All of these 'spiritual behaviours' are intrinsically concerned with transcendence because they are orientated towards an attending to that which is beyond one's own confines. Such behaviours have been evidenced by a further two studies, namely Granstrom (1985) and Baines (1984), to have positive effects on those individuals who engage with and display them in their lives. These beneficent outcomes included carers achieving a more optimistic outlook and a heightened sense of order and coherence about the stressful experience of caring for a partner with dementia.

The conceptual flaw in such studies is that they seek to identify behaviours that are specifically 'spiritual' purely because they evidence a transcendent quality towards that which is beyond the person. Yet, if spirituality is inclusive to all of the human condition then it must also be inclusive of all human concerns, actions or omissions – intra-personal, interpersonal and transpersonal. In this way, the person who faces a cancer diagnosis may be quite still, body language belying inner trauma, chaos and crisis. Yet when a person engages with such themes it evidences spirituality as we have described it in this chapter because it is a seeking to make some sense of an illness that threatens all those elements that bring ballast, meaning and constancy to life – that may even bring death. In essence, this striving to make sense of the diagnosis is congruent with the role spirituality plays in personality integration, and a sense of harmony and meaning in life. Nevertheless, such vibrant semantics again seem out of keeping with the experience of being confronted by such shocking news.

If spirituality is concerned with personality integration, harmony and a search for meaning then the diagnosis of cancer clearly places barriers before the person who seeks to balance these elements. As such, the term 'spiritual distress' can be used to describe the individual's feeling of disharmony, loss of meaning and sense of disconnectedness (Smucker, 1996). Such thinking is consistent with the literature were a lack of meaning has been described as a spiritual crisis (Kierkegaard, 2000). Moreover, Kendrick and Robinson (2000) add that a loss of hope and human contact also fits the defining features of spiritual distress.

The lived experience of spiritual distress often leads a person suddenly diagnosed with cancer to ask the initial question 'Why me?' Such searching is a most natural response when seeking to make sense of situation that is, to all intents and purposes, without sense. Answers to such questions are seldom found; of course, the natural history of the cancer could be explained but causative themes hardly begin to offer a response to this essential question that cuts to the person's very core. The search for meaning cannot offer answers to the question 'Why me?' In essence, the process is often resolved with yet another question 'Why not me?' For if cancer is something that confronts the human condition then our inclusive state means we cannot seek exclusivity from disease. Yet, the realisation that cancer merely confirms the fragility of humanness does nothing to quell the existential plight that its presence brings to the sufferer. We do not use the word 'sufferer' here as a term restricted to corporal pain; the person with a new diagnosis of cancer may not have experienced any physical distress. Yet the trauma of such news can leave a person feeling as though mind, body and soul are being tormented and tortured in unison – cancer playing both roles with ease. In this respect, the malignancy has an insidious presence that thrives by stealth and the demise of healthy tissue. When viewed in this way, such an assault on the human condition readily lends itself to the term 'spiritual distress', were, as we have said, the complete inclusiveness of the human condition is compromised.

What is emerging here is that spirituality is more than a search for purpose and meaning because it embraces additional transcendent elements that move the individual to reach out beyond the concerns of the self. Here we are placing a deliberate emphasis on moving beyond concerns of the self rather than merely transcending the self because we acknowledge that it is impossible to quantify where the limits of the self actually lie. Such notions have implications for the schema of spirituality as it trans-lates to the relationship between the nurse and the person who is newly diagnosed with cancer. This is a particularly relevant and resonant point given the results of recent research that suggests the spiritual distress experienced by cancer patients may be under-addressed by health profes-sionals owing to time constraints, lack of confidence in effectiveness, and role uncertainty (Kristeller *et al.*, 1999).

If the nature of spiritual crisis is about a loss of meaning, sense of disharmony and disconnectedness then a vital focus for the nurse is to offer a professional presence and attendance that engages with these themes. In saying this, we are aware that such language paints broad strokes about the nature of spiritual crisis in a person who has been told they have a malignancy. However, in the clinical experiences of both authors, the concepts found in the literature to define spiritual distress mirror the reactions of individuals having been told they have cancer.

Caring, Transcendence and Hope

Caring can be described as the beneficent attending of one person, through actions or omissions, toward another. Within a nursing context, such themes reflect a transcendent dynamic that moves one person to express a sense of attitudinal relatedness to another. In this way, the mode of caring is evidenced in transcendence through the extending of self for the good of another. This is also linked to the relationship between spirituality, action and the synthesis of meaning. For example, to care for a person who needs a drink of water cannot be evidenced until such a need is acted upon and met. The dynamic of transcendence is evidenced here as the orientation to care through the provision of the water – within this, the action facilitates the creation of meaning. who needs a drink of water cannot be evidenced until such a need is acted upon and met. Conversely, if a person requested a drink and was told by the nurse 'I care for you' in isolation from action, then meaning would lack transparency since this orientation to care was not evidenced by a response that met the need for water.

This relationship between transcendence, care and meaning is poignantly illustrated by the writing of Lyall (1997) who describes a desperately frightening and lonely episode during her stay in hospital because of an acute and life-threatening illness. In one passage, it is night time and Lyall is feeling particularly distressed and isolated; she is unable to articulate her feelings because of the technology that is keeping her alive. Reaching out her hand to a nurse for reassurance, she was brusquely told to go back to sleep and her hand placed firmly back on her abdomen. Contrary to her previous experience of nurses, Lyall comments that this nurse appeared to perceive the nature of caring solely in terms of monitoring the machines that were supplying the drugs that were keeping the patient alive:

> I was grateful for the [nurse's] vigilance. But my spirit needed keeping alive too; I needed to be literally in contact with the pulse of a living being ... As I lay there, too terrified to fall asleep in case I had another nightmare, I felt something furry brushing against my cheek. It was the teddy bear Andrew had brought back from Canada for me. It symbolised the love and prayers of all those who were concerned for me. I was too ill to be ashamed of getting comfort by cuddling a child's toy; at that moment the teddy was all I had. But touching him was sufficient to calm me down and enable me to get some revitalising sleep.

We have already presented the notion that spirituality is what gives focus to the sum of all the parts that make the human condition. For Lyall, the period of crisis provoked a primal urge to seek reassurance and feel the close physicality of another human meaning. Through transcendence, Lyall extended her self in the search for reassurance from the nurse; this focused on a need for affirmation that reflected the very essence of being a human being: 'my spirit needed keeping alive too'. When the nurse did not respond, Lyall reached towards the teddy bear and found there a transcendence symbol that mirrored the love and prayers of all those people important to her. This illustrates that transcendence moves and extends the self towards the 'other' and can focus upon subjects or objects of a human, animate, inanimate or supernatural state. This poignant description of distress evidently resembles the feeling of disharmony, disconnectedness and loss of meaning associated with spiritual distress. Such themes readily apply to a life-threatening episode where the carer has rejected the cared for and left her to seek spiritual affirmation in the guise of a teddy bear.

A core element missing in the nurse's engagement with Margaret Lyall was an attitude and presence that conveyed fidelity and hope. In essence, there was a lack of faithfulness shown through acts of caring that reassured this acutely ill woman that she was the focus of beneficence. Because of this omission, there was also a commensurate affront to Lyall's chances of grasping futurity in a way that held personal significance. Such expectations have been described as essential elements in the formation of hope (O'Connor *et al.*, 1990). Some commentators have chosen to describe the transcendent elements of care delivery in the following way:

> The covenantal relationship, which promotes trust and mutuality, requires bodily mediation in order for its true value to be appropriated by helped and helper alike. The 'sacrament' of caring is the use of the physical closeness of bodies to a therapeutic end, the overcoming of weakness and the restoration of hope which another human presence makes possible (Campbell, 1984, p.111).

There is much that we can learn through Margaret Lyall's writing and experience that can be translated to the care of a person with a new diagnosis of cancer. To this end, we can offer a caring presence geared towards a therapeutic end that upholds the importance of trust and mutuality as catalytic themes that form the prerequisites of hope. In this way, whatever the person 'hopes' for, we can offer concrete responses that cast futurity in the possible rather than the improbable. Taking this further, for example, we cannot offer an absolute guarantee of cure, but we can give an absolute assurance that everything within our professional focus will be done in the person's best and informed interests. What follows from this should be an agenda that creates empowerment through choice and open dialogue; such elements are defining features of patient advocacy (Kendrick, 1996).

Up to this point we have described transcendence as a defining characteristic of spirituality that extends the self towards another. We have discussed this notion in terms of the delivery of nursing care or its omission. Missing from this discussion is the notion of reciprocity. This element relates to the interpersonal dynamic associated with transcendence. Explaining this further, if a nurse delivers care to a patient then this supports the essence of transcendence as a mode of caring evidenced through the extending of self for the good of another. What has not been described is the nature of any positive dynamic the nurse may receive from the patient; this has been described in the following way by Mayer (1992, p.52): 'Care is seen as something delivered to the powerless from the powerful. There is little awareness in the literature of the patient's capacity to give and thus create a mutual relationship'.

This notion of reciprocation is a core aspect of discussions concerning spirituality and transcendence.

Spirituality and Immanence

The interpersonal dynamic of transcendence is concerned with an extension of the self towards another. When concerned with care, this extension of self is focused on a beneficent attending towards another. As we have suggested, this is an unbalanced equation until we consider what comes back towards the nurse in terms of unsought reciprocation. Jacono (1993, p.192) illustrates these themes of mutuality thus:

> The smile of the previously downcast patient after our 'acts of loving', the thank you of family members for the attention to the little details, and the sigh of satisfaction from patients who have been physically and emotionally comforted by our care are all forms of recognition.

The therapeutic essence of giving care is not a restricted, one-way dynamic; quite simply, in giving, nurses also receive and this is evidenced by the mutuality described in the symbiotic themes shown previously in the quote from Jacono. It may be suggested here that in extending the self to attend upon another, the carer is also cared for and sustained through the elements evidenced in mutuality. If nurses did not experience the freely occurring themes of mutuality and reciprocity the experience of care delivery would be static and sterile. Such elements are not rigorously sought from the nurse; in essence, care is not given in the expectation of reciprocation. The benefits that arise from this dynamic are described by Griffin (1983, p.293) in the following way:

> If we sought any of these things deliberately they might well elude us – as in the search for happiness. They are, if you like, gifts coming from the proper and authentic involvement in a particular institutional role. In other words, the recipient of care gives something to the nurse, or to the extent that this process may not be conscious, is the occasion for the nurse receiving some or all of these things.

What has emerged here is that transcendence occurs when the nurse extends the self to beneficently attend upon another. The response of the patient evidences the human themes of mutuality and reciprocation that enrich the state of being for the nurse. This transmission to the nurse of beneficent and sustaining themes is a process that can be called 'immanence' and suggests a balancing element to transcendence; quite simply, the nurse has extended the self to care for another and this has been reflected back in the themes of immanence described here.

The themes we are exploring here are supported in the literature but also resonate with our lived experience of caring for individuals with a new diagnosis of cancer. None of us can tell how a person will react to the news of being told they have a malignancy; the uniqueness of each human being is that reactions to such traumatic information are as varied as the length and breadth of raw emotions. What we can say is that in giving a caring presence we also receive – in a way that mirrors the dynamic of transcendence and immanence we have discussed here. We do not wish to present an image here of all nurse – patient relationships being idyllic and utopian. For example, if a nurse offers a caring presence to a patient with a new diagnosis of cancer and is met with abuse then it is difficult to see how such themes are sustaining. The conditions of immanence are still met, however, because what has come from the patient can be used for reflection and the experience used for teaching and sharing with others. We also acknowledge that abuse can leave the nurse feeling vulnerable and disenfranchised. This raises the challenging notion that the interpersonal dynamic of spirituality need not always be beneficent. Such themes deserve critical scrutiny but go beyond the realm of this discussion.

Conclusion

This chapter has sought to represent and explore the character, purpose and workings of spirituality in nursing a person with a new diagnosis of cancer. What has emerged is that spirituality is partly concerned with a search for meaning and purpose. This search is most clearly evidenced in the working dynamics of spirituality. We have said that some may seek such insights on the top of a mountain where the majesty of nature liberates insights within the self. Such a process illustrates the themes of transcendence and immanence where the individual has extended the self and been enriched and sustained through an external communion, in this case with nature. The terrifying reality of a new cancer diagnosis, however, does not allow a passive search for meaning but forces the individual into a captive state where every living moment seems to focus upon a host of ontological and existential concerns that crucially engage with the spiritual: 'Why me?', 'What if I die?', 'Will I be in pain?', 'What is the hope of cure?' The response that nurses give to such penetrative questions creates an engagement that meets patients in the throes of spiritual distress.

When spirituality is concerned with the interpersonal, we have explored how actions evidence meaning as defined within context and situation. If this is focused within a dynamic of care then the orientation is conveyed to the patient through beneficent attending. The nature of transcendence here captures an attitude from the nurse that is displayed through semantics and actions. These elements give meaning, context and purpose to the active nature of caring and is the critical essence of the attitudinal presence offered by the nurse to a patient with a new diagnosis of cancer.

We have also argued that nurses receive from patients. This is not a scenario born from a purposeful seeking of mutuality but a dynamic where nurses are also sustained and enriched through that which emanates from the patient. Such notions are powerful because they challenge traditional notions that portray patients as passive and acquiescent individuals who are merely the focus of care delivery. Through this channel of mutuality patients mirror the elements of immanence that enrich the nurse. Such themes are captured in the following piece from the moral theologian, Alastair Campbell (1984, p.107):

> The professional, who is aware of how much he or she gains in support, enlightenment and personal development from helping others, may well feel a greater indebtedness. It is often more blessed to care than to be cared for: and the ability to care is frequently made possible by the understanding and sensitivity of the needy person. Such reciprocity suffuses the relationship of caring with a spontaneity, with a sense of grace which enriches carer and cared-for alike.

Finally, the purpose for critically exploring and describing the character, purpose and workings of spirituality in nursing a person with a new diagnosis of cancer was to present a dynamic that is, for the most part, absent from the epistemological base that informs contemporary narratives. This is illustrated by the lack of literature that attempts to explain spirituality in the context of the nurse–patient relationship – this chapter has attempted to address this omission. This is important because dealing competently with a patient's spirituality signals a nurse's orientation to care for that which the profession has taken ownership of. If this ownership is to be authentic then nurses should be familiar with those defining characteristics that constitute spirituality's critical essence. If such themes do not have relevance or resonance then spirituality should be cast out from the concern and focus of nursing (Kendrick and Robinson 2000).

References

Abiven, M. (1995) The Crisis of Dying. *European Journal of Palliative Care*, 2(1), 25–32.
Allport, G.W. (1937) *Personality: a Psychological Interpretation*. Chicago: Chicago University Press.
Baines, E. (1984) Caregiver stress in the older adult. *Journal of Community Health Nursing*, 4, 257–63.
Campbell, A.V. (1984) *Moderated Love: A theology of professional care*. London: SPCK.

Cassell, E.J. (1982) The nature of suffering and the goals of medicine. *New England Journal of Medicine*, 306, 639–4.

Diamond, J. (1998) *Because Cowards Get Cancer Too*. London: Vermillion.

Emblem, J.D. and L. Halstead (1993) Spiritual needs and interventions: comparing the views of patients, nurses and chaplains. *Clinical Nurse Specialist*, 7(4), 175–82.

Engebretson, J. (1996) Considerations in diagnosing in the spiritual domain. *Nursing Diagnosis*, 7(3), 100–7.

Frankl, V.E. (1978) *Man's Search for Meaning : an Introduction to Logotherapy*. Boston: Beacon.

Granstrom, S. (1985) Spiritual nursing care for oncology patients. *Topics of Clinics in Nursing*, 39–45.

Griffin, A.P. (1993) A Philosophical Analysis of Caring and Nursing. *Journal of Advanced Nursing*, 8, 289–95.

Jacono, B.J. (1993) Caring is loving. *Journal of Advanced Nursing*, 18(2), 192–4.

Jasper, K. (1932) *Existentialism. Philosophy 11*. Oxford: Oxford University Press, p.29.

Kaye, J. and K.M. Robinson (1995) Spirituality among care givers. *Image: Journal of Nursing Scholarship*, 3(2), 218–21.

Kendrick, K.D. (1996) Advocacy in later life: an ethical analysis. *International Journal of Health Care in Later Life*, 1(4), 253–9.

Kendrick, K.D. and S. Robinson (2000) Spirituality: its relevance and purpose for clinical nursing in a new millennium. *Journal of Clinical Nursing*, 9(5), 701–5.

Kierkegaard, S. (2000) *The Living Thoughts of Kierkegaard*. New York: New York Review of Books.

Kristeller, J.L., C.S. Zumbrun and R.F. Schilling (1999) 'I would if I could': how oncologists and oncology nurses address spiritual distress in cancer patients. *Psycho-oncology*, 8(5), 451–8.

Long, A. (1997) Nursing : a spiritual dimension. *Nursing Ethics*, 4(6), 496–510.

Lyall, M. (1997) *The Pastoral Counselling Relationship: a Touching Place?* A Contact Pastoral Monograph. Edinburgh: Pastoral Trust, 7, pp.4–5.

May, R. (1969) *Love and Will*. New York: Dell.

Mayer, J. (1992) Wholly responsible for a part, or partly responsible for the whole? The concept of spiritual care in nursing. *Second Opinion*, 26–55.

McSherry, W. and P. Draper (1997) The spiritual dimension: why the absence within nursing curricula. *Nurse Education Today*, 16, 38–43.

O'Connor, A.P., C.A. Wicker and B.B. Germino (1990) Understanding the cancer patient's search for meaning. *Cancer Nursing*, 13(3), 167–75.

Oldnall, A. (1996) A critical analysis of nursing: meeting the spiritual needs of patients. *Journal of Advanced Nursing*, 23, 138–44.

Ross, L. (1995) The spiritual dimension: its importance to patients' health, well-being and quality of life and its implications for nursing practice. *International Journal of Nursing Studies*, 32(5), 451–68.

Salt, S. (1997) Towards a Definition of Suffering. *European Journal of Palliative Care*, 4(2), 97–107.

Smucker, C. (1996) A phenomenological description of the experience of spiritual distress. *Nursing Diagnosis*, 7(2), 81–90.

Weisman, A.D. and J.W. Worden (1976) The existential plight in cancer: significance of the first 100 days. *International Journal of Psychiatric Medicine*, 7, 1–15.

8

Advancing Practice in Cancer Care Ethics

SIMON ROBINSON and PAULINE DODSWORTH

Nurses do not cure stress but they can help people survive it by establishing a healing relationship and by helping them to mobilise their emotional and spiritual resources. (Benner and Wrubel, 1989)

Traditionally, ethics has tended to look for firm foundations on which to place judgements, no more so than in medical ethics and especially where this involved death or dying. Behind much of this foundationalist search has lain 'grand narratives', predominantly Judaeo-Christian. These have aimed to provide sufferer and carer alike with reassurance about the ultimate meaning to life. Based originally upon key ideas such as the sovereignty of God a series of moral principles have emerged, such as the sanctity of life which form the basis of ethical judgement. This deontological or natural law approach (not exclusively religious) makes it clear that certain principles are right or wrong in themselves.

Alongside this, and partially in response, has grown the consequentialist view of ethics. These argue that no principle is without exception and that the moral good is found through maximising utility, the good end, of any act.

Each of these broad ethical theories has important things to say but neither is capable of sustaining the complexities of ethical situations, especially in cancer and palliative care. Apart from the problem of unexceptional principles the deontological approach is invariably caught up in a power struggle, between the moral principle and the autonomy of the individual, and with that the right to determine personal meaning. Such a struggle reaches epic proportions in postmodern times when the old grand narratives are dismissed as imperialist and ethics become so relative as to be almost a matter of taste.

Consequentialism, meanwhile, cannot avoid sneaking in some underlying view of the good in order to give meaning as to what the good is that should be maximised. In any case it tends to ignore the minority who are not part of that maximisation.

Quite apart from the theoretical problems with both these approaches neither sit well with palliative and cancer care. The two theories tend to encourage the model of ethical decision-making which is individualistic and which sees ethics as 'solving' dilemmas, as if there is a rational solution to all problems. Palliative and cancer care involves responding in a systematic and planned way to a human experience, which is full of complexity. Indeed, within that experience the tension between autonomy and shared understanding of what ethical meaning and response might be are perhaps at their most intense, not least because the experience may involve facing up to mortality, survivorship, personal and physical identity and so on.

In this chapter we aim to do two things. First, we will look at a way of approaching ethics in cancer and palliative care, which gives full value to personal autonomy but is also based on common experience and insights. Second, we will look at the particular ethical issues for cancer and palliative care in the twenty-first century. Throughout we shall use the feminine pronoun, for both patient and carer, as inclusive.

The Principles of Cancer and Palliative Care

Reflection on ethical method and meaning must begin with aims and principles of the care itself. Control of the disease, the symptoms and its causes, and addressing the psychological, social and spiritual problems are the main goals. This involves a concerted effort to achieve the best possible quality of life for patients and their families by a multi-professional team (WHO, 1990). Whether cancer or palliative care, the needs of the patient are paramount, she is always at the centre of treatment, care and other decision-making. The family and to a lesser extent the wider community are important. However, the degree of importance, and consequently involvement, is variable and depends in part on the point in the cancer journey and the dynamics of the relationships.

It is often argued that the care of cancer patients is firmly based in the need for treatment, and rightly so, until a cure is deemed not possible. The main aims of treatment are the prolongation of life and the relief of suffering. The expectation of patients and nurses alike is that treatment should achieve cure wherever possible and the relief of symptoms may follow from the curative treatment. Where cure is not possible the speedy and efficient relief of suffering becomes of prime importance. Here then is the move into palliative care, sometime described as 'low tech, high touch' (Twycross, 1995) as opposed to the increasingly 'high tech' of current cancer care.

The WHO definition states that palliative care:

- Affirms life and regards dying as a normal process.

- Neither hastens not postpones death.

- Provides relief from pain and other distressing symptoms.

- Integrates psychological and spiritual aspects of care.

- Offers a support system to help patients live as actively as possible until death.

- Offers a support system to help the family cope during the patient's illness and their own bereavement (WHO, 1990).

Palliative care is not an alternative to cancer care but is a complementary and vital aspect of any patient's care. What is being addressed here is the idea of best practice within nursing, regardless of diagnosis or stage of disease. If symptoms cannot be cured they should be palliated, disease alleviated and independence maintained for as long as is possible. The isolation of patient or family often felt at the point of diagnosis also needs to be addressed as does the fear and anxiety associated with life threatening disease moving towards a dignified death and support for those who are bereaved.

Ethical Meaning and Care

Response to this depth of care has led ethicists to focus on three alternatives:

- The moral decision-making process. Whatever, the ground of one's ethics the professional should have a method for making ethical decisions.

- Articulation of the principles underlying professional ethical decision making and the care relationship.

- The development of virtues and the underlying virtue ethics approach.

Ethical Methodology

Any professional has to give an account of how she has arrived at a moral decision. Simply to rely on the idea of conscience or intuition is inadequate. Apart from the problems of what either of these two ways of knowing actually means both have a strong affect content and therefore are not accounted for simply. The medico/ethical world is not short of decision-making processes, including those developed by Seedhouse (1988) or Niebuhr (1960). Seedhouse gets closer than most to tying in complex ethical reflection into practical care.

These attempts do however hold several dangers. First, they tend to stress the cognitive function of patient and carer. In cancer and palliative care especially there is a strong emotional element, which will inevitably affect any reflection on ethical meaning. Second, in an effort to be academically respectable and exhaustive about ethical reflection they run the danger of being too complex and so too unwieldy to use in practice. Third, there is a danger of process taking over from the care relationship. Fourth, many of the ethical methodologies actually assume that there are absolute principles underlying the whole process, something, which is precisely at issue.

Operational Principles

Randall and Downie argue for several key operational ethical principles, that is, principles that guide rather than prescribe practice, implied in or emerging from the principles of palliative care:

- beneficence
- non-maleficence
- respect for autonomy
- justice
- utility
- self-development (Randall and Downie, 1999).

The aim of relief of suffering clearly is based in the principle of beneficence – looking positively for the good of the other. This goes hand in hand with the principle of not harming the patient – non-maleficence. The question of utility is there at the macro level, to do with allocation of resources, but also at the micro level in weighing up the risks or burdens against the benefits of a particular treatment. Respect for the autonomy of the patient is fundamental, involving respect for goals, values and choices. This guards against manipulative interventions of whatever, especially important given the high vulnerability of these patients.

As Randall and Downie note such principles are necessary but not sufficient. Putting such principles into practice also requires qualities and skills, which in ethical terms are the virtues. Just as with the decision-making process then there is the danger of unthinking adherence to principles, leading to insufficient attention to the basic level of care and the interpersonal dynamics.

More problematic is the point that such principles are not as clear as Randall and Downie take them to be. The principle of justice, for instance, is still very contentious within philosophy, with meanings ranging from justice as desert to justice as fair distribution. Each of these meanings has its own theoretical support.

Respect for autonomy is entirely unclear. At one level it simply means that the patient's right to make her own decision should be respected. However, does this mean that the person's judgements and final decision cannot be questioned or challenged? The term autonomy itself implies that the patient is actually in a position to make a rational decision. However, the experience of illness frequently affects the capacity to make decisions. As Bridges (1980) notes of crises and moments of transition in life these give rise to disengagement, disidentification (loss of identity), disenchantment, and disorientation.

Behind the idea of autonomy (self-rule) is often the assumption that the person is a rational decision-maker who makes decisions without reference to others. The reality is often somewhat different. Most people are not skilled in articulation about or reflection on moral meaning in their life, not least because it involves affective as well as cognitive aspects. They need another to help them reflect and practice that reflection, in effect to gain the skills of ethical decision-making. Along with skills come personal qualities and this leads to an ethic of virtue.

Virtue Ethics

Virtue ethics in recent years have become more popular through the works of Hauerwas (1983) and MacIntyre (1981). The key idea in virtue ethics is that the ethical meaning is communicated through narrative, and that narratives exemplify not principles *per se*, but the virtues, which make up the good character. The narratives are shaped in the context of community and this becomes the place where the virtues are practised.

In respect of palliative care this has concentrated mostly on care of the dying and the issue of euthanasia. Hauerwas, for instance, notes the needs of the community and the critically important factor of developing trust. Euthanasia and its possibility actually destroys that trust, thus not enabling the development of key ethical virtues. It ultimately takes away the power of the patient, and prevents her from addressing the realties of her life, including the reality of suffering.

The problems with the MacIntyre and Hauerwas approach are:

- it simply ends up with a form of relativism. Moral meaning depends upon the particular community narrative, with no way of finding a common morality with other communities.

- while the development of virtues is important, there still needs to be some consensus about the moral end of those virtues.

Each of these approaches is important then but none is sufficient of itself to provide an effective balance between shared moral meaning and individual freedom in the practice of care.

Patients and staff need to feel confident that they have worked through an ethical meaning which is congruent with the care offered and which all can own and justify. A way of achieving this is through covenant ethics.

Covenant Ethics

What makes covenant ethics uniquely applicable to palliative and cancer care is the fact that it spans three areas: pastoral or medical care, spirituality and ethics. It is common in many nursing texts to see the three taken as quite separate, with different needs and different responses, all be they complementary. However, all three come together in the covenant and its central idea of *agape*, or unconditional love. This provides the ground and attitude of care, the foundation of spiritual awareness and the irreducible moral principle. As we shall see while this has often been seen in Christian terms its is not an exclusively Christian idea.

In all this agape provides both the process of care and ethical decision-making and the guiding content. This process and the way in which the different elements come together can best be viewed in the light of the following simple framework:

(a) Enabling the ethical narrative.
(b) Reflection on ethical meaning.
(c) Enabling change.
(d) Empowerment.

Enabling the Ethical Narrative

Faced by the experience of cancer or terminal illness the patient needs primarily to feel accepted. May (1987) notes that the idea of the covenant – derived in his writing from Old Testament examples of covenant agreements – provides this basic unconditional care. The covenant is promissory, donative and inclusive. In palliative care it is critical in the care of the particular patient. When faced by the possibility of major, possibly disfiguring physical change, or by approaching death the patient can easily see herself as 'odd' or 'different', as someone who others are embarrassed to be with, or actually fear to be with. At the heart of this can be a sense of shame that wants to hide the effects of the illness, or approaching death, from the other – even the family. Agape involves *fidelity* to the other whatever her appearance, whatever the response and however bad the patient feels. Love in this sense is not based on the attractiveness of the other but on an appreciation of the other for her self. As Nouwen (1994) notes, this is a love that is communicated in the faintest of glances, assurance of touch, and one which communicates that the carer will still be there tomorrow morning.

May contrasts this covenant with its 'first cousin' the contract. A contract is more specific and conditional. When one of the parties breaks the terms of the contract then the other is freed. Not so the covenant, even when one party is unable to fulfil the contract the other remains in the relationship of care.

There is behind this a more fundamental point about the self-awareness of the patient. The faithful presence of the other enables the patient to begin to see her self and the truth of her situation and in turn to be able to come to terms with that situation, and accept herself in that situation. In effect this involves the development of spiritual awareness. A great deal has been written about spirituality in recent years and we do not have the space to develop this. However, spirituality can be summed up as:

- An awareness of the other – including the self, the other (person or group), the environment and the deity. Any one of these may form the ground of faith in its broadest sense.

- Appreciation of, and the capacity to respond to the other.

- The development of life meaning based upon this awareness. This life meaning then is not simply cognitive awareness, but also affective and somatic awareness.

Spirituality then is not to be equated with religion in any crude way, though religion of course involves a particular expression of spirituality. It is clear however, that spirituality is not a static awareness but one that involves reflection and growth. Hence, if spirituality and the subsequent life meaning are to be sustained there is need for ritual and disciplines which enable reflection and affirmation.

Key to spiritual awareness is empathy. The concept of empathy has of course been claimed as a counselling skill, through the work of Carl Rogers. In fact it is a much broader life skill. Max Scheler describes empathy as involving transcendence, 'a genuine reaching out into another person and his individual situation, a true and authentic transcendence of the self' (Campbell, 1984). This dynamic involves moving away from the things which concern or obsess the self, such as fear or guilt, and which block an openness to the other. It is a natural, unselfconscious awareness that does not hold to 'personal dignity'. As the patient experiences the faithfulness and empathy of the carer so she is enabled to gradually reveal different aspects of the self. This revelation in the context of a caring and secure relationship enables her to become more aware of herself. This gradual revelation of the self comes through the development of the person's narrative. Articulation of her narrative, but especially in relation to the experience of her illness enables the patient to begin to own her basic life meaning. It is also a way of developing reflection and thus testing the narrative. As she articulates her story so she too, perhaps for the first time, is the listener. She may become aware of feelings, which have not been expressed before, or of important values or people which she has taken for granted. She may become aware of the foundation of faith which as Fowler (1996) notes is critical to any sense if identity and life meaning, be that in family, belief system, religion, environment and so on. In turn then the patient begins to develop empathy, for herself and others.

The awareness, which emerges from this reflection, is anything but simple. Indeed, as Heinz Kohut (1978) notes, such empathy has at its heart the acceptance and holding together of ambiguities and inconstancies. At the core of such ambiguities is the awareness of the self as both the same as and different from others. Many, for instance, are afraid to articulate the emotions of fear or shame because they feel that others do not experience it. To admit they felt this would make them different and strange. For the patient awareness of the self as both dependent and independent also struggles to be held together.

Many things stop the development of an empathic narrative of truth, from fear to lack of reflective practice, to the felt need to project guilt or bad feeling on to others. Hence, the presence of the carer has to be skilled in reflecting back the narrative as she hears it developing, thus helping the patient to hear. The continued presence of the carer enables this truth to be tested and accepted. Indeed, such truth can only be received through a care which reassures the value of the other whatever is revealed.

What emerges then is a narrative of emerging truth about the self, others and the situation. This is only possible through the covenant presence of the carer, enabling an holistic awareness, principally through the acceptance of empathy.

It is precisely this pastoral and spiritual relationship which provides the basis for moral meaning.

Ethical Reflection

The covenant ethic is in one sense very general. The principle of agape does not tell you specifically what to do in any situation. Nonetheless, agape does provide substantive operational meaning and also enables ethical dialogue, which develops and sharpens, shared ethical insight.

First, the ethic of agape involves *inclusive* care for others. Bauman (1993) argues that this is precisely the starting point of any ethical attitude, that we take responsibility for the other. In reflecting upon the Holocaust he notes that many of the experts who were involved in the war machine fulfilled several moral obligations – to client, workforce, etc. – but that the basic commitment to fellow humans was exactly missing. They perceived the other as purely different – with no sense of common humanity. This therefore must be the starting point in moral reflection. How that responsibility is to be worked in detail is what follows. Bauman stresses that this attitude is pre-rational, in the sense that it cannot be based on any rational calculation, such as Rawl's view of fairness. Viewed in calculative terms it does not 'make sense' to accept responsibility for the other.

Second, agape generates a series of secondary principles. The stress on inclusive concern, seeing the other as part of humanity, leads to the principle of *fellowship* or *community*. These in turn lead to the principles of *participation* and *mutual responsibility*. Concern for the particularity of the other leads to the principles of freedom and *diversity*. The concern for the other also leads to the principle of *equality of respect* and other forms of equality.

Third, just as the spiritual attitude and awareness of agape holds together the different, often ambiguous, aspects of the person, so agape the basic moral principle holds all these subsidiary principles together. Without this, such principles could easily become polarised, not least in the political game of freedom versus equality.

Fourth, the very fact that agape holds different principles together in tension demands that the person takes responsibility for her own ethical response. It is not possible to slavishly apply a principle. The person then becomes her own moral interpreter.

Fifth, agape provides the moral criteria with which any principles can tested. Any moral principle can be used to bad ends without this. Freedom by itself, for instance, can be used to encourage a view of moral meaning which is individualistic and not inclusive. The principle of self-sacrifice can easily be used to oppress and marginalise groups such as women, if it does not hold to genuine inclusiveness, that is seeing the self as having the same needs as others.

Agape also guides the process of developing moral meaning, not least in the way that it enables value clarification. This is not a simplistic value clarification which accepts that whatever the person thinks or feels is right. Agape in enabling the person to articulate her narrative brings to the fore all the different elements of moral meaning. Sometimes these have already been thought through and the narrative reaffirms them. However, even familiar moral meaning can be severely tested by the experience of a crisis. For instance, the father who has refused to speak to his son for many years because he revealed his homosexuality may in the light of a crisis begin to re-examine why he holds such views and what values are more important to him. The mother who has spent 30 years working for her four sons and in a marriage that is increasingly loveless may begin to re-examine her view of the family and of her own identity faced with breast cancer. As the life meaning is examined in the light of the crisis many will find that their life meaning has been chosen by them or for them at an early age and that their ethical principles are built upon injunctions and feelings of shame, which they have no control over. As Kaufman (1980) notes in his work on shame, if the person is to develop control over her spiritual and ethical life it is important to return such shame to its origins. All of this confirms that moral meaning does not simply operate at the level of concept and rational discourse, but is radically affected by our emotions and thus out life history (Robinson, 2000). Such emotions affect how we view moral principles and how we use them, to good or bad ends.

In all this the agapeic presence of the carer enables the person to see the different ethical meaning in the narrative and to see the contradictions and conflicts which emerge. As Halmos (1965) reminds us, when these kinds of ambiguities and contradictions arise a patient or client may well fell anxious. It is not the task of the carer to 'solve' that problem or to ease the anxiety. On the contrary, the carer must allow the person to handle the apparent conflicts of the narrative. This may mean simply holding together the different aspects, such as sameness and difference, or it may mean choosing to develop a different approach to life – developing different ethical values.

This clarification of values continues in the development of dialogue between different ethical narratives in the person's life. We are all immersed in different ethical systems throughout our life – family, school, workplace, church, etc. As we reflect on the network of relationships that make up our life meaning, so the different relationships will bring conflict and contradiction which sets up the need for dialogue about the different ethical ideas. This is a perfectly natural way of testing what we do think and how our values actually operate in the different parts of our life. It is precisely such dialogue which begin to enable shared moral meaning, a meaning which emerges from the increased awareness of the other, through their values, awareness of what is the same about their values and what might be distinctive. As we shall see in the next section, establishing such meaning develops further around response to the particular situation.

Agape is involved in this dialogue both as facilitator and as one of the narratives. Indeed the caring relationship itself embodies the agapeic covenant. The patient will come to know something about that through the experience of empathy and through testing the care of the other, something which is naturally done in any caring relationship (Robinson, 2000). Such an experience of inclusive care then provides criteria for reflection on the different narratives. The religious narrative which stresses honouring parents, for example and which can easily be used to generate guilt, can be tested against the principles of community and freedom. Importantly, such an ethical principle is not threatened by the testing of agape. Rather is the central meaning revealed, and the principle strengthened through such dialogue and testing.

The development of ethical meaning around the therapeutic relationship can also lead to short-term 'contracts', articulating what is expected from carer and patient and which in turn can be the basis for further reflection and renewal of ethical and spiritual awareness.

Enabling Change

The agapeic ethic is by definition transformative, developing awareness of the self and others, and with that developing the capacity to respond to the other. Central to this transformation is, first, the strengthening and development of *integrity* and, second, the development of *shalom*.

Integrity is a virtue or a collection of virtues, which is ultimately about the person being at peace with herself. Solomon (1992) suggests that these virtues come together to form a coherent character. Integrity involves:

- Making connections between the different aspects of the self (cognitive, affective and physical) and between self and practice. This leads to holistic thinking, and integration of the different aspects of the self – cognitive, affective and somatic.

- Consistency of character, between the self and its values and practice; past, present and future; and different situations and contexts.

- Honesty. This involves a high degree of transparency, with the person open to the other.

- Responsibility. This involves taking responsibility for meaning and value. Without this there is not real ethical thinking, simply the acceptance of cultural norms, or lack of them.

Human limitations make it impossible to have complete integrity. It involves rather a continual process, with the person discovering and rediscovering more about the different aspects of the self and how they affect each other. Hence it is impossible to speak of achieving wholeness, but is possible to speak of being at one with the self in and through continued growth and renewal.

This sense of peace is extended to the relationship with the other in the development of shalom. This Judaeo-Christian concept has often been used to translate such different ideas as peace, health, welfare, etc. It is not about a static peace, but rather the development of right relationships – relationships which themselves have integrity. Hence it is not an easy peace, but one that also involves justice, in the sense of facing up to wrongs in any relationship. At the heart of this is the constant transformation of relationships embodied in forgiveness and reconciliation. This, of course, is often at the heart of the patient's experience. Faced by the shadow of death and often the challenge of her belief systems there is the felt need to 'put things right'.

Establishing right relationships is a proactive and interactive activity, which moves naturally from the development of awareness of the other and the self. As the other is known so sameness as well as difference emerges and the possibility of forgiveness and reconciliation emerges. As Smedes (1993) notes, forgiveness itself is based upon the acceptance of common humanity, common failings, common needs and common possibilities. The change which agapeic ethics enables then is not simply of the individual person but is essentially relational. This contrasts sharply with Joseph Fletcher's situation ethics, which sees agape as the base of what is simply utilitarian calculus. Shalom is rather about the quality of the relationship.

Inevitably the individual and relational transformation which is enabled through agape leads to questions of responsibility. Faced with different relationships and different needs how is patient or nurse to respond and how is the responsibility to be shared. The empathic reflection outlined above first, begins to build up a picture of an awareness of the limitations of the person herself, what she can and cannot do. Second, as this is shared in the light of the different situation and the different capacities of others involved this naturally moves into negotiation of responsibility. Finch and Mason (1993) from their work with families note that negotiation is critically important for development of moral meaning. Their work found that the majority of families that had to reflect on who would take responsibility for another member of the family, for example ageing parents, did not refer to moral rules or principles. They rather spent time on negotiating and renegotiating how responsibility might be shared. This very process enabled the development of shared moral images which themselves became the ground for commitment and continuity, despite the lack of formal ethical vocabulary. This established a 'moral reputation' and in turn moral identity with person's 'constructed and reconstructed as moral beings'.

All this directly affects the quality of ethical decision-making. Being aware of others and their needs and also seeing them as resources in sharing responsibility actually leads not so much to a maximisation of utility as to an increase in possibilities, and to the building up of relationships. This involves what used to be termed stakeholder analysis – looking at all involved, what power they have and how they can work together for shared ends. Better decisions are made, because more people are involved in reflection and outcome.

This working out of purpose and the way in which it can be fulfilled is also important to the development of life meaning. Such meaning is made up of two parts; knowledge of acceptance of the self, and knowledge of purpose and contribution to others. The covenant enables the person to feel valued for the self alone, and so to have faith in the self and others. The ethical response enables the person to feel valued for contribution to the community, to others. Tawney (1994) can thus sum up spiritual well being as, 'finding one's work and doing it'.

The negotiation of responsibility then leads to the further shared moral meaning, generated through collaborative response to need. At one level then the meaning comes through practice. Such shared practice confirms and develops trust. This extends to the detailed planning and collaboration in putting plans into effect. The covenant then has ultimately to be embodied – in relationships, contracts, organisation, structures and so on.

Habermas (1990) suggests that there might be rational rules drawn up for this kind of discourse. However, useful though they may be, it is important to note that they cannot work without the underlying agape. It is precisely such an ethic which is required if what Habermas sees as the political and personal constraints to discourse are to be overcome and if the difference which emerge in any discourse are to be handled creatively.

An Ethic of Power and Freedom

As the person begins to develop or confirm her ethical identity so is there a deepening of her own power. This is fundamental to the covenant ethic. As Vanstone (1977) notes love gives away the 'power to determine the issue of love, its completion or frustration, its triumph or tragedy'. All the nurse can do is to wait and hope that the other will reveal and respond, just as the father of the Prodigal Son, waited, having given his son all that he needed (Luke 15: 11–32). Scheler notes of empathy that openness to the other is not possible if there is any attempt to dominate or manipulate. There is no room for the 'top down' approach of previous generations of nurses resulting in a paternalistic model of care.

The nurse gives the patient what she needs, through attention and time so that she can begin to articulate her narrative. By giving her the support and presence to handle the contradictions and difficulties which emerge from that reflection, by remaining committed whatever may emerge or however strange or different the person may feel.

If the person does not wish to enter into the covenant of care that is her right. However, what emerges from this is a rich, complex and far more satisfying view of freedom:

- freedom to express and hear the self;

- freedom to test and dialogue, and hence freedom to learn. This acknowledges the point that learning is critical to the development of the person. The covenant in effect sets up a continual learning cycle;

- freedom *from* oppressive ethics and injunctions which may have ruled the life, note least any conditional ethics;

- freedom to establish the basic identity in faith relationships;

- freedom to accept realities about the self, others and life situations;

- freedom to embody the ethical response.

Respect for autonomy, which simply seeks to avoid being oppressed, has little to commend itself, especially when the patient is assailed by the doubt and difficulties of the experience of cancer or of the fact of impending death. Such a view of autonomy also assumes that the rational person has already worked out their position and it must not be changed by others. This is to present a false picture of the person, as someone who has nothing to learn. By definition the person is constantly being asked to learn. Moreover, whilst respect for the other demands that she is not manipulated this does not preclude challenge. On the contrary the non-judgemental challenge which is part of open dialogue with others and with different value systems is a critical part of developing individual and group value systems. Far from threatening autonomy, this strengthens moral identity, increases moral confidence, and in turn improves autonomy.

The development of this moral freedom then involves both negative freedom (freedom from) and positive freedom (freedom to). At its heart is the development of freedom as capacity, in effect the development of the virtues.

We have already considered the importance of *empathy* and *integrity*. These and other ethical virtues are developed precisely in the dynamic of the caring relationship which enables the person to articulate her narrative and to reflect critically on, and with the different stands of, that narrative. Equally important virtues for patient and staff alike are faith, practical wisdom and hope (Robinson, 1997).

Covenant ethics then is fundamentally social and dialogic. Dialogue enables the development of individual moral identity. It also strengthens shared principles by focusing on their real meaning, and enables the development of moral meaning by collaborative response in practice. The agapeic covenant provides both consistency and constancy, by providing grounds for trust in the dialogue and providing important moral criteria. Hence, the ethic embodies both constancy and change, a concern for both *community* and for *freedom*, and provides the basis for dialogue between both content and process and theory and practice.

Future Challenges

Ethical issues have always been an important part of healthcare for a variety of reasons, although not always articulated clearly by nurses and rarely discussed openly with patients. Palliative care ethics, and perhaps to a lesser extent cancer care ethics, have become stuck in a small number of fundamentally traditional areas, namely to treat or not to treat, the euthanasia debate, autonomy, etc. But as new concerns are raised new questions are asked and new answers need to be found. We are living through exiting times. As medical technology advances and 'breakthroughs' are discussed almost every day in the media, it results in treatment regimes that are more complex and radical, the balance of benefits and burdens become more difficult to assess and public expectations are raised. There seems to be an increasing belief that there is an answer for everything, a clear link with other already-discovered factors and a belief that doctors can prolong life and postpone death almost indefinitely. For example, pneumonia was historically seen as the 'old man's friend'; today, and since the development of antibiotics, there is an expectation that no one will die from a 'simple' infection. This of course is untrue. On the other side of the debate people who are wary of modern technology and fear a prolonged and undignified death hold different concerns. This leads to a highly emotionally charged environment in which healthcare is delivered and nurses may find themselves in a conflict of roles based on the potential clash between their personal ethical values, belief systems and their professional concern for the vulnerability of the patient and his family.

Changing Attitudes to Death and Dying

Along with this is the change that has occurred in the social meaning of death for most western cultures and peoples attitudes to cancer, death and dying. For example, many people until they have to confront their own death, will have had a very limited experience of any form of dying. However, it must not be forgotten that as our society becomes increasingly diverse in its cultural mix that this can not be presumed to be true for all people. This is in contrast to previous generations where death was seen as an ever-present part of life and people were generally closely involved in family dying, at the very least. So for the most part death has little or no place in peoples' day-to-day existence any more. There is of cause a paradox here for as death has become increasingly removed from our day-to-day lives it has become an omnipresent event in the media. It is often portrayed in very graphic detail and as such although often very distressing in nature it has further lost some of its previous meaning and proximity. It is something that happens to others. This necessitates nurses having to consider how their patients, family carers, and they themselves may respond to death and dying. They need to recognise the tensions that may exist between the approach adopted by those who are trained to deal with death, that is, the professionals, and lay perspectives. And also how this may influence how they may frame the decisions they make in respect of care delivery and the need to be present along side patients and their families. This can only be done effectively by encouraging the development of the narrative.

Resource Implications

Another potential area of conflict is related to demographic changes, which cannot be ignored, as we move into an unprecedented era of increasing numbers of elderly people who not only live longer but may also have different expectations of healthcare professionals from previous generations. These expectations are of better health and an increasing number and variety of readily available services that will facilitate this longevity. As statistically it is known that the longer a person lives the greater the probability of them developing cancer this adds to the demand on cancer and palliative care resources. Assuming that resources in healthcare are finite, and moreover that healthcare rationing is now explicit, how can the distribution of these scarce resources be easily resolved? Add to this the issues of earlier diagnosis and all that this entails, the ever-escalating cost of new and more radical treatments and, because of more active treatments, the increasing need for prolonged aftercare, how can the purse strings ever stretch far enough?

The issue of cost is always on the agenda and by its very nature the cost of cancer care and palliative care is very demanding of resources. Cancer care and treatment costs escalate almost daily as new research findings lead to new treatment regimes, and the call for palliative services to be made available to an every increasing number and diversity of patients also results in stretched resources. Add to this the difficulties associated with the assessment and audit of 'value for money' in these arenas and the complexity of the dilemma becomes evident, particularly in palliative care where outcomes are primarily qualitative and therefore seen as being far less measurable than curative cancer treatments and survival rates. It could be argued that the important, and seemingly simple question, is how much are we prepared to pay through our taxes to provide all that is deemed necessary to facilitate care for these groups of patients. Even if, as Whynes (1997) states, there is evidence to suggest that the general public is prepared to pay more than was previously expected, there are still the perspectives of service providers and policy-makers to be taken into consideration.

Resources are not only monetary, and along with finance there must also be considered the scarcity of expertise. Currently, approaching ten years after the Calman-Hine Report (1995) in the United Kingdom, cancer services are still, in some areas, without appropriately qualified professionals and equipment. Add this to the national shortage of nurses in all disciplines, and particularly in specialist areas of care, and the ethical challenges to be considered in providing not only adequate care, but best care for these patients increases daily. This then poses the key question as to who are the appropriate practitioners to care for cancer and palliative care patients and their families. Increasingly patients are cared for in their own homes by their families with the support of community nursing and social care staff. These are not only patients who are reaching the end of their lives but are also those receiving radical courses of cancer treatment either at home or as day patients. Should care only be given by 'skilled workers' and who are these workers and what specific skills do they need? If in part the philosophy of palliative care is concerned with the comfort and quality of life of patients then it could be argued that generic skills, particularly those of families, rather then specialist skills are needed along with human skills such as empathy. But the same cannot be said of situations where specialist skills are definitely needed to meet the needs of cancer patients undergoing treatment regimes that often result in onerous side effects and require complex and individual care plans. However palliative care addresses more and more the rehabilitation needs of patients, as it seeks to help them achieve and maintain their maximum potential, even if this has become limited due to the progression of the disease. Perhaps here it is less easy to argue for highly specialist skills as what is being addressed is truly 'best' care, individual care – something that all practitioners should be striving for with all patients. So how are decisions to be made as to where the money for training should be spent? Should most resources be put into developing quality pre-registration programmes, at whatever academic level, or is it more fruitful to educate more and more highly specialised nurse practitioners? But decisions surrounding the education of professionals should no longer be left to the service providers and the educators alone; as the needs of patients and clients change, they as consumers should be increasingly involved in the development of educational initiatives.

Survivorship

Other challenges to face are those associated with the phenomenon of survival. Until recently the words cancer and survival were rarely included in the same sentence. Today more and more people are surviving cancer as a result of earlier and better diagnoses and improved treatments and care, so as this population increases we need to consider what survival means to the individual. Although it is acknowledged that there is an increasing number of cancer survivors, little seems to have been considered as to what their long-term needs and fears might be. In fact, the literature seems based on the biomedical model of health and illness (Quigley, 1989; Welch-McCaffery *et al.*, 1989) rather than a consideration of the enduring problems of survivorship. The general understanding of the word survivorship is associated with the aftermath of living through a catastrophic life event (Breadon, 1997). How true for cancer patients and their families! Some survivors talk of experiencing nightmares and flashbacks to treatment; is this not akin to post-traumatic stress syndrome, suffers of which receive aftercare. Others live their entire life with altered body image or changed functioning, the constant fear of reoccurrence, never free of suspicion, and the struggle to return to 'normal', to become again a father, a lover, a worker, after long periods of being a patient, an invalid and oft times a passive recipient of care. A new issue for this population is the possibility of a second primary tumour developing after survival from the first cancer – a 'side-effect' of longevity. Many survivors speak of the guilt attached to survival when others have not been so 'lucky'. Women who survive breast cancer to then be told it has been identified as the type of cancer that has genetic links also experience guilt surrounding the legacy that they may have given her daughters. Do nurses have the skills to meet these new and complex needs? Do we currently have the ethical frameworks to support decision-making for advocating appropriately for these people? For example, how would nurses use to the satisfaction of both nurse and client the more traditional approach to ethical decision making when a client is faced with the prospect of prophylactic bilateral mastectomy? Practice can no longer hover on the edges of paternalism but must move wholeheartedly into partnership.

Frank (1991) describes the experience of some survivors as having a feeling of separation between mind and body, that one of the tasks of survivorship is the regaining of a sense of wholeness and becoming one again in body and mind. One survivor, Joan, cited in Breadon (1997), talks of '... so they fixed the body and the rest is left to me'. So often in practice the fragmentation of care occurs. But after treatment the body can never return to its previous state. The person, no longer the patient, has again to move towards an acceptance of self, but a new and altered self. Should she be left to achieve that alone or does the nurse have a contribution to make? If the nurse does have a role to play, then this approach to care demands a faithfulness and unconditional acceptance of others (patients and their informal carers) even when the person is no longer receiving formal care. It necessitates time, an acknowledgement of limitations, both of resources and self, which are often disturbing and painful to achieve and especially to sustain. Currently it could be argued that people are 'dismissed' at the point of discharge as they are seen to be cured, they no longer have any physical problems, and are therefore no longer our responsibility. To identify the needs and expectations of this group of people we maintain should be approached through allowing the development of the narrative but it takes time, insight, commitment and ultimately money to consider how these needs might be met. So should survivors of cancer and its treatment be offered aftercare and for how long should this continue? As Joan alluded to, the 'fixing' of the body remains the overriding objective of professionals, but the fear, anxiety, guilt, etc. are left to the patient to address. Having developed a therapeutic relationship with a patient while undergoing treatment, the nurse could extend this to the provision of psychological care and support in the period following discharge from the care of the oncologist. The nurse alone may not always best achieve this. Working with other members of the multidisciplinary team, for example a psychologist, would not only deliver care which is firmly based in the philosophy of cancer and palliative care, but also enable the patient to further reflect upon and reconsider their spiritual self and how this new situation can impact upon a new life. This could be achieved through the development of 'short- term' contracts that are frequently redefined as the survivor moves forward. But this of course brings us back to the issue of resource allocation and the dilemma of who should receive which care and can after care be justified for some when others are waiting for initial treatment? There is a debate here around whether other statutory and/or voluntary organisations could be involved in the further care of survivors. The latter, particularly, would seem to be one way forward, in line with changes over recent years in health and social policy to increase the community dimension of care.

Conclusion

Whether working with cancer patients undergoing active treatment or patients with palliative care needs, the principles of care remain constant. They centre on the importance to continuous meaningful communication with the person and family, to provide appropriate and effective symptom control when necessary; to respond appropriately to their ongoing and changing needs and to provide effective liaison and the sharing of information between professional and lay carers. In short, the development of relationships which themselves have integrity where the development of trust is paramount and the nurse as well as the patient can negotiate responsibilities and has knowledge of the acceptance of the self and a knowledge of her purpose and her contribution to others. This is where the idea of covenant ethics is so important. It demands faithfulness and unconditional regard, an acceptance based on an appreciation of others as individuals, identifying what their needs and expectations might be and looking for ways in which they might be met in collaboration with others. And in an ever-changing healthcare environment recognising that these collaborations may often be with groups and individuals not previously considered.

Two things might be levelled against this ethic and its use in cancer and palliative care. First, it seems yet another set of professional skills has to be learned, adding yet more to the tasks of the nurse. Second, the process of the narrative, reflection, value clarification, responsibility negotiation and practice might appear over-long. To the first we would answer that the skills and qualities which are needed by the nurse are not as such specialist skills. Empathy as, noted before, for instance, is not so much a specialist counselling skill, as a basic human/spiritual skill or quality. As such it underlies many other skills areas, not least in diagnosis. What is critical is that the nurse and the care team should value such virtues, and thus reinforce their development in each of the members of the multidisciplinary team.

Such virtues are equally important to the patient; a good example is hope. People need hope to be sustained, hope is part of the essence of life, part of what might be defined as the spirituality of a person. For many patients and their families, the diagnosis of cancer or the decision that their future care will have a palliative focus rather than one which strives for cure robs them of that much needed hope. It is as though their future has been taken away from them, as if there is nothing left to live for – they have been delivered of a death sentence. Of course this is not the view that all people have, as some are able to grasp the challenges ahead and retain hope throughout the cancer journey. But what of those who find hope difficult to maintain? Do nurses have a role in restoring and maintaining hope or is this the realm of the clergy? As with many other areas of healthcare today, the boundaries are blurred and nurses are able to work as agents of hope when they work closely with their patients and consider decision-making as part of the covenant with that patient. We need to recognise the sameness as well as the differences in the skills of the two disciplines. Both the professional spiritual adviser and the nurse have no need to develop special skills but have to begin to negotiate how the 'spiritual expert' can work with the 'nursing expert' to best meet the needs of the patient. Their skills are the same but are also different, different that is in the intention of the 'expert' and the expectations of the patient. The patient who is most active in the early hours of the morning will turn towards the person who is present, the nurse. It must also not be forgotten that the process of the narrative, reflection, responsibility negotiation, etc., take time and the patient will chose who, for her, is the right person with whom to explore these issues. The nurse is able to provide empathy, presence and time for reflection, reflection that is cognitive as well as affective. There is need for assessment and reassessment, a partnership that is constantly developing not only with the patient but with the other members of the team, always open to review and modification just as the hopes of the patient need to be reconsidered as the agenda changes. Sometimes it is sufficient to be a hopeful person, to have hope invested in others, not just hope of recovery but hope based upon achievable goals – goals which are real and not idealised. The attitude of hope informs and contributes to further decision-making, enabling a person to be creatively open to possibilities and also accept genuine constraints (Robinson, 2000). The presence of hope restores a sense of empowerment.

As to the process this is less important than the presence. It is the presence of the nurse as an individual and in a team that enables the moral and spiritual meaning to be articulated and shared. This may involve all the aspects of reflection and negotiation noted above. It may involve but one meeting where the patient is searching for and ready for that presence, and thus is given space to articulate her feelings and hopes, and to affect her reconciliation.

But when a man says to his fellow man, 'I will not let you go. I am going to be here tomorrow waiting for you and I expect you not to disappoint me', then tomorrow is no longer an endless dark tunnel. It becomes flesh and blood in the brother who is waiting and for whom he wants to give life one more chance. ...Let us not diminish the power of waiting by saying that a life-saving relationship cannot develop in an hour. One eye movement or one handshake can replace years of friendship when man is in agony. Love not only lasts forever, it needs only a second to come about. (Nouwen, 1994)

References

Bauman, Z. (1993) *Postmodern Ethics*. Oxford: Blackwell.

Benner, P. and J. Wrubel (1989) *The Primacy of Caring*. Menlo Park, CA: Addison-Wesley.

Breadon, K. (1997) Cancer and Beyond: the question of survivorship. *Journal of Advanced Nursing*, 26, 978–84.

Bridges, W. (1980) *Transitions: Making Sense of Life's Changes*. Menlo Park, CA: Addison-Wesley.

Calman, K.D. and D. Hine (1995) *A Policy Framework for Cancer Services*. London: Department of Health.

Campbell, A. (1984) *Moderated Love*. London: SPCK.

Finch, J. and J. Mason (1993). *Negotiating Family Responsibilities*. London: Routledge.

Frank, A. (1991) *At the Will of the Body: Reflections on Illness*. (Boston: Houghton-Mifflin.), cited in K. Breadon (1997) Cancer and Beyond: The Question of Survivorship. *Journal of Advanced Nursing*, 26, 978–984.

Habermas, J. (1990) *Moral Consciousness and Communicative Action*. Oxford: Polity Press.

Halmos, P. (1969) *The Faith of the Counsellors*. London: Constable.

Hauerwas, S. (1983) *The Peaceable Kingdom*. Notre Dame, IN: University of Notre Dame.

Kaufman, G. (1980) *Shame The Power of Caring*. Cambridge Shenkman.

Kohut, H. (1978) The Psychoanalyst in the Community of Scholars, in P. Ornstein (ed.), *The Search for the Self*. New York: International University Press.

McIntyre, A. (1981) *After Virtue*. London: Duckworth.

May, W. (1987) Code and Covenant or Philanthropy and Contract, in S. Lammers and A. Verhey (eds), *On Moral Medicine*. Grand Rapids: Eerdmans.

Niebuhr, R. (1960) cited in V. Tschudin (1994) *Deciding Ethically*. London: Bailliere Tindall.

Nouwen, H. (1994) *The Wounded Healer*. London: Darton, Longman & Todd.

Quigley, K. (1989) The adult cancer survivor: psychosocial consequences of cure. *Seminars in Oncology Nursing*, 5, 63–9.

Randall, F. and R.H. Downie (1999) *Palliative Care Ethics*. Oxford: Oxford University Press.

Robinson, S. (1997) Helping the Hopeless. *Contact*, 127, 3–11.

Robinson, S. (2000) Agape and Moral Meaning in Pastoral Counselling. *Journal of Pastoral Care*, 54(2), Summer.

Seedhouse, D. (1988) *Ethics: The Heart of Health Care*. Chichester: Wiley.

Smedes, L.M. (1993) Stations on the Journey from Forgiveness to Hope, in E.L. Worthington Jr (ed.), *Dimensions of Forgiveness*. Philadelphia: Templeton Foundation Press.

Solomon, R. (1992) *Ethics and Excellence*. Oxford: Oxford University Press.

Tawney, R.H. (1994) *Commonplace Book*. Cambridge: Cambridge University Press.

Twycross, R.H. (1995). *Introducing palliative Care*. 3rd edn. Oxford: Radcliffe Medical Press.

Vanstone, W.H. (1977) *Love's Endeavour, Love's Expense*. London: Darton, Longman & Todd.

Welch-McCaffery, D., *et al.* (1989) Surviving adult cancers: Part 2: psychological implications. *Annals of International Medicine*, 111, 517–23.

Whynes, D. (1997) Costs of Palliative Care, in D. Clarke, J. Hockley, and S. Ahmedzai, (eds), *New Themes in Palliative Care*. Buckingham: Open University Press.

World Health Organization (1990). *Cancer Pain and relief and Palliative Care*. Technical Report Series 804. Geneva: WHO.

9

Withdrawing Treatment: Ethical Issues at the End of Life

JANET HOLT

For a patient with an incurable disease, the goals of care have been stated as the alleviation of suffering, the optimisation of quality of life until death occurs and the provision of comfort in death (Cherny, 1996). The notion of dying well is of importance to all of us and of particular significance to healthcare professionals specialising in palliative care. Advances in technology and the availability of new pharmacological and surgical treatments means that for some patients a range of treatment options may be open to them. For patients, recognition of their ability to participate in decisions about their care and treatment is a concern illustrated in a recent report published by Age Concern. The report identifies 12 principles of a good death, which include 'to be able to retain control of what happens' and 'not to have life prolonged pointlessly' (Debate of the Age Health and Care Study Group, 1999). However, because of the nature of the disease, not all patients are able to retain control, and decisions have to be made by others involved in their care. This chapter will examine some of the ethical dilemmas that arise when decisions about discontinuing treatment have to made in cases when patients are capable of making decisions themselves, and when decisions have to made by others involved in their care. The concept of autonomy, living wills, definitions of treatment and what constitutes acting in someone's best interests will be considered in the context of professional practice in palliative care.

Respecting Autonomy

Everyone is entitled to decide what should and what should not happen to them and patients can expect to have the decisions they make respected. The ethical justification for this is explained by the principle of autonomy. Derived from Greek, autonomy literally means self-rule but is

a concept difficult to define precisely. Beauchamp and Childress (1994) suggest that autonomy has acquired meanings as diverse as self-governance,
liberty, privacy, individual choice and freedom of will. Despite the different
interpretations, the autonomous person can generally be considered to be
free from the controlling influences of others and from limitations that
restrict meaningful choice. The autonomous person therefore 'acts in accordance with a self-chosen plan', while a person with diminished autonomy is
'at least in some respect controlled by others or incapable of deliberating
or acting on the basis of his or her desires and plans' (Beauchamp and
Childress 1994, p.121). Even people who are deemed to be autonomous
may have temporary constraints placed upon them affecting their freedom
of choice and diminishing their autonomy. Harris (1985) suggests that
defects in the person's ability to control their desires or actions, defects in
reasoning, defects in the information available and defects in the stability
of the person's desires diminishes autonomy. Just to recognise that a person
is autonomous or capable of making rational autonomous choices however,
is not enough. The person must also be respected as an autonomous agent,
that is someone with a right to hold views, make choices and to decide
upon a course of action based on personal values and beliefs. As health professionals we can at best, 'provide people with the conditions of autonomy,
and help then attain or at least not stand in the way of the fulfilment of
their autonomously made choices' (Soifer, 1996, p.42).

Respecting personal autonomy is an important principle for health
professionals and forms the basis of the law governing consent. This is
recognised in *The Code of Professional Conduct* (UKCC, 1992) where nurses,
midwives and health visitors are advised to work collaboratively with
patients and clients, foster their independence, and recognise and respect
their involvement in their care. However, respecting autonomy absolutely
may not always be practical and there are often other issues to be taken
into consideration as well as the wishes and desires of the patient. In many
cases, controversy does not arise. The patient is aware of their diagnosis,
prognosis and whatever treatment, if any, is available. They discuss the
options with the health professionals and come to a decision that all
parties agree is the best way forward. The patient has made an autonomous
choice, and the health professionals have no difficulty in respecting that choice.
But other situations are not so straightforward and conflict may arise
between the patient and health professionals involved in their care. A
patient may be competent to make an autonomous choice, but the
decision they make is one with which the health professionals have more
difficulty. Suppose that some form of treatment is available and recommended by the health professionals, but the patient refuses it, or alterna-
tively, the patient insists upon receiving treatment not recommended by
the health professionals. Should the patient's choice be respected in such

cases? While respecting someone's autonomy is an important moral principle, it should be recognised that it is not the only moral principle that needs to be taken into consideration. Nor can autonomy be considered to be an absolute moral principle, that is one that will take precedence in every case, as a persons autonomous choice will be legitimately constrained by the rights of others. For example, a patient may decide that their life is not worth living and ask a nurse to help them die either by administering a lethal injection or by providing them with appropriate drugs to commit suicide. Even if the nurse was convinced that the patient's autonomy was not diminished and that they had made a rational choice, it does not follow that in order to act ethically and respect their autonomous decision, the nurse must comply with the patient's request. The patient may have a self-chosen plan upon which they wish to act, but in doing so, they are asking the nurse to act unlawfully, and appealing to respecting the principle of autonomy would not be a plausible defence. In this situation the nurse must also make an autonomous decision. She may of course agree to the patient's request and accept the consequences of her actions, or she may choose not to. Whatever course of action the nurse decides upon will need to be made on the basis of her own autonomous decision and not because she is obliged to act according to the patient's wishes. Respecting autonomy is therefore a prima facie right, that is, one that must be fulfilled unless it conflicts with an equal or even stronger claim. In this example, the nurse's claim that she must act within the law would be stronger than the patient's claim that they should have their autonomy respected.

Futile Treatment

Other situations may arise where the patient insists on being given treatment not recommended by the health professionals. The patient understands that there is very little chance of the treatment being beneficial, but they decide that they wish to be given it anyway. If we are to respect the autonomous wishes of the patient then treatment should be given, but in doing so the health professionals may question whether or not they are acting in the best interests of the patient if the treatment is futile. If respecting the patient's autonomy is the most important ethical principle, then giving the treatment is justified. It may be the case that the best interests of the patient are indeed protected by allowing the treatment to be given, but such a decision needs to be balanced with other competing demands such as practising according to best evidence and appropriate utilisation of resources. An important aspect of the recent reform of the National Health Service (NHS) was the establishment of the National Centre for Clinical Excellence (NICE). In *A First Class Service* (DoH, 1998), it is argued that patients suffer if resources are not used effectively, and one of the functions of NICE is to assess existing and new interventions for both their clinical effectiveness and cost-effectiveness.

Clearly, administering treatment that is both costly and ineffective cannot be of benefit to society as a whole or to the individual patient. Even ardent supporters of the sanctity of life argument recognise and agree that there are some circumstances when not administering treatment is morally permissible. The philosophy of palliative care begins with the recognition that cure is not possible; that the emphasis of treatment should change from cure to care and that death should not be postponed (Jones, 1995). The British Medical Association (BMA) has addressed this issue directly in its guidance on making decisions about withholding and withdrawing treatment: 'Unless some other justification can be demonstrated, treatment that does not provide net benefit to the patient may, ethically and legally, be withheld or withdrawn' (BMA, 1999: p.1).

Farsides (1999) considers the term 'net benefit' in this context is significant and useful. Rather than suggesting that the person's life is not worth living, the value of the treatment is assessed. The benefits and burdens of administering treatment are examined enabling decisions to be based upon whether intervention or continued treatment is justified. There is nevertheless some dispute regarding what constitutes medical treatment and whether the administration of nutrition and hydration falls within this definition.

Nutrition and Hydration: Treatment or Care?

In the 1993 case *Airedale NHS Trust* v *Bland*, the House of Lords did not draw a distinction between the provision of food and fluids by artificial means and medical treatment, and held that tube feeding was part of the regime of treatment and care (Kennedy and Grubb, 1994). The BMA (1999) follows this and other legal judgements and classes the use of nasogastric tubes, percutaneous endoscopic gastrostomy and total parental nutrition as medical treatment that may be withdrawn in some circumstances. This definition of feeding as medical treatment is however, not universally accepted. While acknowledging that health professionals are under no obligation to provide medical treatment with a view to simply prolonging life, Gormally (1995) argues that this does not extend to omitting to feed the patient. Gormally draws a distinction between the duty to provide medical treatment and the duty to provide ordinary care such as food, fluids, warmth and shelter. While it may be reasonable to withdraw medical treatment such as antibiotic therapy, it is not reasonable to withdraw ordinary care such as tube feeding from the patient. Health professionals are under a duty to always provide ordinary treatment. Wright (1993) challenges the judgement in Bland as a betrayal of nursing values and maintains that feeding patients, however artificially, is a fundamental aspect of nursing therapy. This view is upheld by Keown (1997) who makes a distinction between administering futile treatment and considering a life to be futile. Quoting Dr Keith Andrews, a leading authority on persistent vegetative state, Keown argues that the only reason that tube feeding was classed as treatment was so that it could be withdrawn. The House of Lords condoned this action because it believed that the patient's life rather than the treatment was futile and there was therefore a need to find some way of ending it. The ruling in *Airedale NHS Trust* v *Bland* has also been reconsidered in light of The Human Rights Act which came into effect in the UK on 2 October 2000. The Human Rights Act incorporates provisions from the European Convention on Human Rights into UK law, and Article 2 of the convention guarantees a right to life. Applications had been made on behalf of two women, each diagnosed as being in a permanent vegetative state, to withdraw artificial nutrition and hydration. The request to discontinue feeding was granted and Dame Elizabeth Butler-Sloss who presided in the case ruled that the principles laid down by the House of Lords in the *Bland* case were not affected by this new piece of legislation and therefore not incompatible with the human rights convention.

The provision of nutrition and hydration does appear to be part of nursing care and to fail to administer fundamental human needs may seem to be an abrogation of nursing duties. Because nutrition and hydration are necessary for life, it is assumed that they are a requirement for a comfortable death also. Welks (1999) examines whether administering fluid in the end stages of life are necessary to alleviate suffering and concludes that numerous studies have shown that providing hydration is not absolutely essential for comfort and may even cause discomfort. Kennedy and Grubb (1994) suggest the solution to the dilemma of whether nutrition and hydration form part of medical treatment does not lie in the process of labelling interventions, but in remembering that health professionals are obliged to act in the best interests of the patients. In some circumstances this means that patients should be allowed to die, a decision that some patients can and will make for themselves.

Being in Control

If a competent person refuses to eat or drink, do health professionals have an ethical or legal duty to ensure that the nourishment and fluids are given? Suppose that Peter, a 48-year old man suffering from motor neurone disease for many years, has increasingly become dependent on others to help him with hygiene and nutrition and hydration. After some consideration, Peter decides that his life is not worth living and he begins to refuse all nutrition and hydration. Peter's carers are clear that his decision, albeit one with which they are not fully in agreement is rational and autonomous. They understand that they can comply with Peter's decision and not give him food or drink, or they can override his decision and administer nutrition and hydration by artificial means and force-feed Peter. It may be argued that Peter has in effect made a decision to commit suicide and that it is morally and legally questionable for any health professional to allow this to happen and not intervene. As far as Peter is concerned, the law is quite clear on this issue. Under the terms of the Suicide Act 1961, the right to suicide is recognised; however, assisting someone to take their life by aiding, abetting, counselling or procuring the suicide of another is an offence. In Peter's case, he does have a right to take his own life, but his disabilities mean that he is restricted to exercising his right in a negative form by refusing nutrition and hydration. While it is unlikely that the health professionals would be liable to prosecution for aiding Peter's suicide, force-feeding him against his will would almost certainly be open to charges of battery or assault. The intentional touching of a person without consent constitutes the tort of battery, and a patient whose valid consent has not been obtained can sue in the civil courts for compensation. In some cases a criminal prosecution for assault may also arise (Fletcher *et al.*, 1995).

To act morally, the health professionals must resolve the dilemma of not intervening and respecting Peter's autonomous decision, or paternalistic intervention and administering nutrition against his will. There is a pragmatic approach to solving this issue concerning the practicalities of actually administering nutrition and hydration to a person without their consent. If the patient is conscious, it may be an impossible task, but a decision not to feed Peter needs to have clearer and more robust reasons than simply saying that its not practical. If the health professionals are convinced that Peter's decision was as autonomous as possible and that his autonomy was not compromised, for example using Harris's (1985) criteria, then they can ethically justify respecting his wishes by appealing to the principle of autonomy. Furthermore, it may be argued that they are morally obliged to do so. To override Peter's autonomy would be to act paternalistically, that is believing that it is right to make a decision for someone without taking into consideration that person's wishes, or even to override their express wishes (Fletcher *et al.*, 1995). The health professionals may believe that they are acting in the best interests of Peter by administering nutrition and hydration even though it is against his will, in an attempt to save his life. Whether the health professionals' belief to be acting in Peter's best interests is sufficient to justify paternalistic intervention is open to scrutiny. Unless Peter's autonomy is diminished, it implies that the health professionals know better than Peter himself what is best for him. Ethically, to override a competent person's autonomous decision is a difficult position to sustain, and a belief to be acting in the person's best interests is alone an insufficient reason for overriding his autonomy. This was also the opinion of The House of Lords Select Committee on Medical Ethics that state in its report: 'We strongly endorse the right of the competent patient to refuse to consent to any medical treatment for whatever reason....no member of the healthcare team may overrule the patient's decision' (House of Lords, 1994: para. 234).

Towards the end of life, not all individuals are able to make their wishes known and decisions have to be made by the health professionals in conjunction with the patient's family and friends. In some cases, the patient will have made their wishes known in advance in discussions with involved in their care, or in writing in the form of a living will.

Living Wills

Living wills were proposed by lawyer Louise Kutner in 1969 and introduced in the United Kingdom by the Voluntary Euthanasia Society in the 1980s. There is some confusion in the use of terminology as the terms, advance statements, advance directives and living wills are used interchangeably. The term 'living will' appears to be the most familiar with the general public, although official documents and discussions in legal cases tend to use the term 'advance statements' or directives. Drawing up a living will gives individuals an opportunity to express their preferences to others, particularly health professionals if they are unable to communicate them verbally. They are documents which 'allow a person to state the criteria on which they would wish treatment to be given should then become incapable of making their own decisions' (McHale *et al.*, 1997).

It is not possible to know how many people have drawn up a living will, but recently published research indicates that although many people are unaware of living wills, once informed of the subject, they are interested to hear about them (Schiff *et al.*, 2000). When preparing a living will, the person should make their preferences known in a clearly written statement. Specially designed forms can be obtained from organisations such as the Voluntary Euthanasia Society, The Patient Association and The Terrence Higgins Trust. While there is no statute in the UK governing living wills, their use is recognised in common law, that is, law made by the judges who adjudicate in different cases. The BMA has also published a code of practice to guide health professionals in the use of advance statements in clinical practice (BMA, 1995). In 1997, the Lord Chancellor's Department published the green paper *Who Decides*, seeking opinion, among other things, on the Government's proposal to legislate on living wills. Following the consultation period, a decision was made not to take forward legislation on living wills. The Lord Chancellor drew attention to the fact that advance statements have full effect in common law, but considered it unsound to fix into statue a set of rules when the case law influenced by medical advances was still evolving. The guidance contained in the case law together with the BMA's code of practice was deemed to provide sufficient flexibility to determine the validity and applicability of an advanced statement (Lord Chancellor's Department, 1999). This means that health professionals are obliged to respect the wishes of the patient regarding which treatment they would like to receive or reject as set out in their living will.

> Competent, informed adults have an established legal right to refuse medical procedures in advance. An unambiguous and informed advance refusal is as valid as a contemporaneous decision. Health professionals are bound to comply when refusal specifically addresses the situation which has arisen (BMA, 1995, p.5).

It is important to note that the person drawing up the living will is free to change their mind while still competent to do so and either discard the document or make changes to it. While only applicable to appropriate and lawful requests, there are still many advantages to making a living will. Patient autonomy is recognised and it gives an opportunity for dialogue with healthcare professionals about treatment options when drawing up the document. A written expression of the patient's desires gives guidance to those making decisions when dilemmas arise and the patient is no longer capable of being consulted. There are also disadvantages to consider. Young healthy people may not be able to predict how they will see things such as illness or incapacity in the future, and judgements may be based upon misunderstanding. While care may be taken to be as specific as possible in the document, the actual clinical situation may not match the circumstances identified in the document, which could make it even more difficult for health professionals to resolve dilemmas about treatment. An example of this would be a broad statement 'no reasonable prospect of recovery', which may be interpreted by different people in different ways. There is also always the possibility that new treatments may become available that had the patient been aware of, they would have wanted to receive (Samuels, 1996).

The difficulties of writing and interpreting living wills should not be minimised, but they do have an important place in clinical practice. Increased understanding and awareness of their function accompanied by research into their use and effectiveness will enable living wills to be of benefit both to patients and those caring for them at the end of their lives to ensure that death is how they should want it to be.

Acting in the Patient's Best Interests

Many patients in the final stages of their illness will be able to make their wishes known, and have ensured that all those involved in their care are aware of their preferences. Others will be unable to communicate or not had an opportunity to discuss their needs, and will not have drawn up a living will. Decisions about care and treatment in these circumstances will have to be made by those caring for them. Health professionals must act in the best interests of the patient and will probably seek the opinions of those closest to the patient to inform their decisions. This may not always be a straightforward process. There may be conflict between differing groups of health professionals regarding the best course of action, relatives and friends may disagree with the health professionals or even with each other about what they consider the patient would have wanted. Recourse to the law in these situations will probably not help resolve the dilemma. In law, no one is able to give consent on behalf of an adult, so consent from a relative is unnecessary and would carry no force in English law. The legal responsibility for any decisions therefore lies with the treating doctor and in particularly difficult or contentious cases, a legal opinion can be sought. This does not mean that others involved in the care of the patient should not be consulted, as to do otherwise would scarcely be considered good practice, and healthcare professionals are expected to involve relatives in any decisions that are made regarding the patient's treatment and care. The UKCC (1992), for example, advises nurses to work in an open and co-operative manner with patients' families. Furthermore, palliative care extends further than the patients themselves to encompass achieving the best quality of life for patients and families, and offering a support system to those close to the patient during the illness and subsequent bereavement (Gilbert, 1996). The duty placed upon healthcare professionals to act in their patients best interests is a theme running through all codes of practice, advisory documents from professional bodies and texts on healthcare ethics. Determining the course of action to be taken may not simply be a matter of clinical judgement, but may also encompass an ethical judgement. While the BMA (1999) acknowledges that decisions taken in the best interests of the patient are likely to be influenced by subjective responses, Kuhse (1997) claims that the twin requirements of such ethical judgements are that they must be impartial and supported by reason. This means that decisions should be made fairly and upheld by a satisfactory justification for the course of action to be taken.

Rachels (1993, pp.13–14) makes this point well in his description of the conscientious moral agent:

> Someone who is concerned impartially with the interests of everyone affected by what he or she does; who carefully sifts facts and examines their implications; who accepts principles of conduct only after scrutinising them to make sure they are sound; who is willing to listen to reason even when it means that his or her earlier convictions may have to be revised; and who, finally, is willing to act on the results of this deliberation.

While this description of the moral agent is not exclusive to ethical dilemmas in healthcare, it appears to be particularly relevant to the complex situations that arise when caring for dying patients, their families and friends. Decisions about withdrawing nutrition and hydration may be particularly difficult for the family to make. White and Hall (1999) discuss the role of family members in making decisions about withholding treatment and withdrawing treatment and conclude that although both actions have the same ethical significance, deciding to withdraw nutrition and hydration may cause more psychological and emotional anguish than deciding to withhold it. Eating and drinking are symbolically significant activities, and a causal connection may be made between a decision to withdraw nutrition and hydration and the patent's subsequent death for which family members may feel some responsibility. Conflict of any sort between health professionals and relatives is undesirable and should be resolved, but if this is not possible, the health professionals' duty to act in the best interests of the patient is the stronger claim. It is difficult to argue that administering futile treatment to a patient is morally acceptable simply on the grounds that a relative has requested it. Health professionals must act in the patient's best interests, and an inability to communicate the preferred course of action to the relatives should not be confused with making a morally correct decision on the part of the patient.

In palliative care, healthcare professionals are challenged by ethical dilemmas, many of which centre on decisions to discontinue treatment and may be of a complex nature. The importance of respecting autonomy is well recognised in modern healthcare and is a recurring theme in advisory documents produced by professional bodies as well as forming the basis of the law relating to consent. Ideally, patients will be full participants in decisions about their treatment and care, and can expect their wishes to be respected even if their preferred course of action is not one recommended by the healthcare professionals. Nevertheless, in some circumstances the decisions will need to be made by others involved in their care. There appears to be an increasing awareness of the role of living wills in assisting healthcare professionals to make judgements on behalf of those no longer able to do so for themselves, and their recognition in common law is established. Despite being potentially beneficial, the use of living wills is not as yet prevalent in clinical practice and decisions will still need to made on behalf of patients without their preferences being known. In these circumstances, healthcare professionals are obliged to act in the best interests of each individual patient in accordance with guidance from professional bodies and with regard to the law. Participation in end-of-life decisions is fraught with ethical dilemmas for healthcare professionals but such decision-making constitutes an important aspect of palliative care to ensure that whenever possible the principles of a good death can be put into practice.

References

Beauchamp, T.L. and J.F. Childress (1994) *Principles of Biomedical Ethics*. 4th edn. New York: Oxford University Press.

British Medical Association (1995) *Advance Statements About Medical Treatment*. London: BMA.

British Medical Association (1999) *Withholding and Withdrawing Life-prolonging Medical Treatment*. London: BMJ Books.

Cherny, N.I. (1996) The problem of inadequately relieved suffering. *Journal of Social Issues*, 52(2), 13–30.

Debate of the Age Health and Care Study Group (1999) *The Future of Health and Care of Older People: the best is yet to come*. London: Age Concern.

Department of Health (1998) *A First Class Service*. London: Department of Health.

Farsides, B. (1999) Withholding or withdrawing treatment. *International Journal of Palliative Nursing*, 5(6), 296–7.

Fletcher, N., J. Holt, M. Brazier and J. Harris (1995) *Ethics, Law and Nursing*. Manchester: Manchester University Press.

Gilbert, J. (1996) Palliative medicine: a new speciality changes an old debate. *British Medical Bulletin*, 52(2), 296–307.

Gormally, L. (1995) Walton, Davies, Boyd and the legalisation of euthanasia, in J. Keown (ed.), *Euthanasia Examined*. Cambridge: Cambridge University Press.

Harris, J. (1985) *The Value of Life*. London: Routledge.

House of Lords (1994) *Report of the Select Committee on Medical Ethics*. London: HMSO.

Jones, E.J. (1995) Hospice and Palliative Care, in F.A. Huser (ed.), *Palliative Care and Euthanasia*. Edinburgh: Campion Press.

Kennedy, I. and A. Grubb (1994) *Medical Law Text with Materials*. 2nd edn. London: Butterworths.

Keown, J. (1997) Restoring moral and intellectual shape to the law after Bland. *The Law Quarterly Review*, 113, 481–503.

Kuhse, H. (1997) *Caring: Nurses, Women and Ethics*. Oxford: Blackwell.

Lord Chancellor's Department (1999) *Making Decisions; The Government's Proposals for Making Decisions on Behalf of Mentally Incapacitated Adults (CM4465)*. London: The Stationery Office.

McHale, J., M. Fox and J. Murphy (1997) *Health Care Law*. London: Sweet & Maxwell.

Rachels, J. (1993) The *Elements of Moral Philosophy*. 2nd edn. New York: McGraw Hill.

Samuels, A. (1996) The Advance Directive (or Living Will). *Medical Science Law*, 36(1), 2–8.

Schiff, R., C. Rajkumar and C. Bulpitt (2000) Views of elderly people on living wills: interview study. *British Medical Journal*, 320(7250), 1640–1.

Soifer, E. (1996) Euthanasia and persistent vegetative state individuals: the role and moral status of autonomy. *Journal of Social Issues*, 52(2), 31–50.

UKCC (1992) *Code of Professional Conduct*. London: UKCC.

Welk, T.A. (1999) Clinical and ethical considerations of fluid and electrolyte management in the terminally ill client. *Journal of Intravenous Nursing*, 22(1), 43–57.
White, K.S. and J.C. Hall (1999) Ethical dilemmas in artificial nutrition and hydration: Decision making. *Nursing Case Management*, 4(3), 152–7.
Wright, S. (1993) What makes a person? *Nursing Times*, 26(89), 42–5.

Part III

The challenges facing nurses who seek to advance practice in cancer and palliative care are considerable. However, there are now unprecedented opportunities for nursing to have a significant and sustained influence on the development of services that will make a real difference to those living with cancer. The authors in this section address the critical success factors in the achievement of improved care through the advancement of nursing.

Taking an international perspective, Chapter 10 explores the evolution of advanced practice in nursing. In changing healthcare systems, where there is a recognition of the potential of nursing, there is a need to clarify several key issues. That is, to determine educational standards and competencies of advanced practitioners within specialist domains. It also requires that professional boundaries are challenged and revised. For example accepting and exercising full prescriptive authority will be a major area of development for advanced practice nurses in the United Kingdom. These are huge challenges but essential in order to make advanced practice a reality. Chapter 11 also recognises opportunities for nurses and sees them articulated through the health policy agenda. Nurses are exhorted to inform and influence that policy. Advanced cancer and palliative care nurses must rise to this challenge.

Issues of management, leadership and service development in cancer and palliative care form concluding chapters in this section and in the book. These issues of course are central in moving services forward and advancing the profession. This centrality becomes apparent in the chapters. A vision for leadership is offered in Chapter 12, which focuses upon the achievement of influence through commitment and emotional connection. The notion of leader as 'helper' or 'servant' is offered as a sustainable model suitable, indeed essential, in times of great change and turmoil. The final chapter examines the development of specific health policy in cancer and palliative care and its implementation in one region in the United Kingdom.

Part III

10

Making Advanced Practice a Reality: An International Perspective

JEAN STEEL

Specialisation is a mark of the advancement of the profession. The purpose of this chapter is to discuss the use of terms related to advanced nursing practice and specialisation. A specific comparison will be made between the United States and the United Kingdom. These two countries have taken the leadership in describing their standards for advanced practice within a larger framework of all nursing. While the taxonomy of advanced practice differs in both countries, there are commonalities that permit the continuing evolution of the profession. Differences have occurred because of national healthcare policy and academic structure and systems. Comparing the countries' interpretation of advanced practice and specialisation will set the stage for a discussion of philosophy. The professional scope of practice and the standards which guide nursing's practice will be used to further the argument that advanced practice *is* a reality. While a brief discussion of advanced practice for cancer nurse specialists will be presented, it is by no means a complete discussion of how advancement occurs within the field. Using the philosophies of both countries and beliefs about advancing the profession, the individual practitioner in a specialty such as cancer or palliative care will be energised to further the specificity within their field.

Terminology can be viewed as shifting sands. It moves with the tide, expanding or restricting boundaries and is influenced by a variety of factors, beliefs, traditions and knowledge. The terminology of advanced practice and specialisation has been validated by a host of professional societies and official bodies. Similarities in definition appear in the worldwide literature, most particularly in the United Kingdom and in the United States. Interpretations of roles appear somewhat different, depending on situation, interest and available resources. Interpretations influence direction or movement in role development and are affected by educational and clinical standards and patient needs.

In the United States, advanced practice has evolved from a variety of role titles and a conceptualisation of what the practice represents. In 1992, the American Nurses Association (ANA) defined advanced nursing practice as: nurses who conduct comprehensive assessments, demonstrate a high level of autonomy and expertise in the diagnosis and treatment of complex health problems, using the resources of individuals, families and communities and identifying the actual and potential health problems. Nurses in advanced practice use clinical decision-making to integrate education, research, management and consultation into their clinical role and function in collegial relationships with nursing peers, physicians, and others who influence the healthcare system (ANA, 1992). Later, the Association clarified that the term 'advanced practice' was to be used to refer exclusively to advanced clinical practice. This would include practitioners who had earned a masters degree in a clinical area, rather than a functional area such as administration, teaching and research (ANA, 1995).

Nurses in advanced clinical practice thus have to possess an earned masters degree in an area of clinical nursing. The roles that were described as advanced practice included clinical nurse specialist, nurse practitioner, nurse anesthetist and nurse midwife. Within each of these roles, the nurse performs basic nursing interventions in addition to new therapeutic strategies for actual or potential health problems, illness prevention, wellness care and provision of comfort. Specific elements of advanced practice include a greater depth and breadth of knowledge (ANA, 1996), collection and management of data, development of care plans and implementation of treatment plans.

At the time of the ANA definition of advanced nursing practice in 1992, advanced practice nurses had a variety of educational preparations. Those without masters degrees were considered to have met the educational requirements for advanced practice (ANA, 1996). They were 'mentored', or 'grandfathered' into the level of advanced practice. Since that time, the profession has moved to establish entry into advanced practice by way of masters level of education. By 1996, there were 161,711 nurses in advanced practice (DHHS, 1998) and by 2000, a modest estimate of 200,000 qualified as advanced practitioners. This represents 6 per cent of total nurses in the USA. Entry into advanced practice roles, therefore, has been determined to be by masters degree in nursing. While there has been significant discussion regarding this qualification, most national and state regulatory bodies have accepted this determination.

In the UK, the UKCC in 1994 defined the advanced practice nurse as practitioners who were changing the boundaries for the development of future practice, they were pioneering and developing new roles responsive to different needs and were advancing clinical practice, research and education, thus enriching all of professional practice (UKCC, 1994a). The advanced practice nurse was seen as stretching professional boundaries in the delivery of care and pioneering new roles as determined by public need. They also included a significantly new focus on influencing national policy (UKCC, 1997).

While no position has been taken officially regarding educational standards for entry into advanced practice (now referred to as higher level practice by the UKCC), a variety of efforts seem to lead toward this development. Universities across the UK are offering masters programmes for the study of advanced or higher level practice.

In 1998, McGee described nurses in advanced practice as being on the cutting edge of the profession, moving previous boundaries outward and providing leadership to the whole of the profession. McGee stated that, due to the lack of standardisation in practice and consensus in definition, advanced practice has not yet emerged in understanding and implementation (McGee, 1998b). Others noted the components of the practice would include an integration of practice, education, leadership, research and consultancy (Elliot, 1998) and depend heavily on individual characteristics of the professional (Davies and Hughes, 1995). The UKCC (1994b, 1997, 1999) further described the work of the advanced level nurse as advancing clinical practice, research and education and fostering new roles that would reflect changing needs and finally, influencing local and national healthcare policies. (Albarran and Fulbrook, 1998).

Specialisation

Like the term 'advanced practice', 'specialisation' within nursing has been described by both professional organisations and legal bodies. Implementation appears to have differing perspectives in the UK and the USA. In the United States, specialisation in practice is seen as a narrowed focus of care. It moves nursing from a homogeneity of clinical interests to a heterogeneity of practice and is seen as a mark of advancement of the nursing profession. Specialisation includes application of a broad range of theories in determining phenomena of concern for the narrowed focus. Further, it includes empirical and controlled research both to clarify particular aspects within the domain of nursing and also to generate change in existing nursing practice. It also expects that practice will evolve (advance) as a result of patient and community needs (ANA, 1980).

As all of nursing has expanded, changing the scope of practice, some nurses choose ways of expanding their intellectual capabilities in particular areas of interest. Movement of boundaries is a consequence of changing technologies, research and changing consumer needs. Thus, the boundaries of the profession continue to change as new technologies and knowledge are applied to the clinical practice of nursing. While the initial meaning of specialty nurse referred to nurses graduating from specialised hospitals or practising as a private duty nurse, the evolution of the term has brought an understanding that specialisation in nursing practice clarifies, revises and strengthens existing practice. It refines practice at a higher level, permitting new application of knowledge from the specialist to the generalist. It could be summarised that advanced practice has to do with the profession's continuing evolution, Specialisation refers to what nurses in advanced practice choose as their narrowed focus of interest.

In the United Kingdom, the RCN in 1988 defined the nurse specialist as experts in a particular aspect of nursing care, who demonstrate refined clinical practice, as a result of significant experience in advanced expertise, and knowledge in a branch or specialty. They further clarified the role of specialty practice as involving a clinical and consultative responsibility, teaching, management, and application of relevant nursing research. The designation of specialist is only applied when the nurse is involved in all of these aspects (RCN, 1988). In 1994, the UKCC stated that the specialist and advanced practitioner had an obligation to achieve a higher level of competence in practice than other nurses in the setting (UKCC, 1994b). Given the acknowledged lack of agreement on measurement of competency, this description is hard to apply. The UKCC did, in 1994, further clarify that the specialty nurse applies high levels of judgement and discretion in their practice and by participating in clinical nursing audit, contributing to research, teaching and supporting professional colleagues (UKCC, 1994b). They added in 1995 that the nurse specialist has a narrowed focus for care, works within a team of care-givers and has managerial responsibilities (UKCC, 1995).

Throughout the UK literature, specialist and advanced practice have been used interchangeably, mingled with specific role titles such as nurse practitioner. Castledine's seminal research described the work of some 353 nurses with the title of clinical nurse specialist (Castledine, 1982). Later, McGee described the work of 320 nurses with a different set of titles, but suggests that the designation of specialist and advanced may be 'artificial' (McGee, 1998a, p.181). Both researchers, however, identified similar components of a role in specialisation with the newer emergence of role titles, such as nurse practitioner. In later work, Castledine (1998) has suggested a framework for a clinical career structure that acknowledges specialty practice based on experience, competence and knowledge. With this structure, additional titles are concretised and made explicit. Goodman defines specialty practice in cancer nursing as nurses who have completed a proscribed educational experience in cancer care and who, on the job, demonstrate skill in rendering care to patients with cancer (Goodman, 1998).

The four areas for initial registration in the UK – adult, child, mental health and learning disabilities – complicates the use of the term specialisation used at a higher educational level. Although there is essential core knowledge within the first years of education, once the specialty is chosen, subsequent completion of the initial registration does not include broad nursing knowledge of all areas of healthcare service. This prevents the beginning practitioner from entry into other generic aspects of practice, thus limiting their future practice options. A generic entry level nurse can only practice in one of these four areas without seeking further education. It appears that this initial choice by the novice nurse makes that nurse a specialist on completion of the pre-registration programme of study. The use of such terms here complicates the national understanding of specialisation. Distinctions between educational specialty and occupational specialty (activity as a result of formal education and long years of practice) are not clear.

Discussion

In the United States, advanced practice in nursing refers to nurses who have acquired the knowledge base and practice experiences to prepare them for specialisation, expansion, and advancement in selected practice roles (nurse practitioner, clinical nurse specialists, nurse midwife and nurse anesthetist) through a formal masters degree in nursing. The specialisation of nursing's practice occurs through the concentration of practice into a specific field or focus. Expansion refers to acquisition of new practice skills (not necessarily knowledge). Advancement includes both specialisation and expansion and is generally characterised by a new integration of theories (knowledge) and skills (ANA, 1995). Thus, to merely expand one's skills is limiting if the knowledge base is not included. Furthermore, to speak of 'expanded practice' alone is dangerous as those skills eventually become expected practice for all members of the profession (Steel, 1994).

A practice discipline, such as nursing, grows, thrives and persists as its practitioners expand or move the boundaries outward. Advancing the profession is caused by new technologies and knowledge applied to the profession by a cohort of nurses prepared to describe, test, refine and implement new approaches to patient problems.

The terms for advanced practice roles, for example nurse practitioner, refer to the role one plays in the clinical setting. It does not define the specialty or body of knowledge used to perform the activity. Thus, the term nurse practitioner is generic as a role. Specific to the body of knowledge, one's title must describe knowledge. Thus, it is appropriate to speak of the primary care nurse practitioner or the acute care nurse practitioner. When used in this manner, the title refers to the role within a specialty. Further, delineation can occur with a 'subspecialty' of particular interest. What is important in the development of advanced practice roles is not to be rigid and specific in titling. It is dangerous to limit the boundaries of advanced practice as it may prematurely shut the borders of practice opportunities. In addition, advanced practice nurses differ in implementation of their new work because of location, interest and need.

In this new millennium there will need to be assurances that the advancement is relevant to the profession, fits within the profession's ability to advance and that it is based on knowledge, not solely on roles. The current debates as to the preeminent role must fade as the professional nurse discovers advancement based on science, knowledge and patient care needs. Characteristics that were once described as advanced, become an expected part of the whole and those specialists move on to discover new strategies, creating yet another cycle of advance. Differentiating between levels and titles may be trivial to the reality of advancement. Protracted debate may slow the pace toward advanced or higher level practice, but may be a necessary feature for the UK as roles of specialist and higher level practitioner and nurse consultant are established and clarified.

The greatest challenge to development of advanced practice nursing is to maintain a balance between nursing's basic practice and beliefs and newly acquired skills and knowledge. Those who do not understand and embrace the concept of advancement may be quick to judge the advanced practice nurse as being outside the domain of nursing. Clearly, the challenge for the practitioner is to maintain a delicate balance of what has been and what will be. When we are uncertain or unsure, we may hold in contempt those who choose to work differently. For example, when the first nurse practitioners in the United States began in the early 1970s, the activity of history-taking and physical examination was considered doctor's work and was severely questioned by professional nurse members. Twenty years later, the activity, responsibility and authority for history-taking and physical examination has become an integral part of pre-registration educational requirements and most nurses now implement the activity as a significant part of expected nursing practice. Likewise, the activity of 'diagnosis' was once a protected responsibility of physicians alone. Through the development of nursing diagnosis, nursing process, and a broadened understanding of the process of 'diagnosis', it has now become an expected part of the nurses' work; in fact, one cannot practice without the ability to diagnose. To use a diagnosis is merely to label, to name or to identify the problem. Our society has expanded the initial use and meaning of the term diagnosis.

In the United States, the advanced practice nurse is prepared in masters level education, not through the review of established practice skills or repetitive practice, but by the synthesis of new knowledge and skills into the existing foundation of nursing's practice. Masters education offers the nurse greater depth, range and competencies, resulting in a broader repertoire of effective solutions for patient need, patient populations and healthcare systems. As a result, the advanced practice nurse is optimally suited for managing more complex, uncertain, and resource-limited situations. This agreement on and commitment to a minimum of masters level education is becoming the norm for higher level practitioners in the UK with the UKCC suggesting that higher level practitioners must be at a minimum of masters level and perhaps PhD level (UKCC, 1999, 2002).

Certain characteristics of the nurse and advanced practice prevail throughout education and practice. These characteristics include common core knowledge (i.e. research and theory), clinically precepted experience (mentoring from experts) and dialogue with appropriate faculty to achieve synthesis of knowledge and skill into advanced practice. The clinical component of advanced practice nursing education at masters level, termed 'the practicum', needs to be a carefully constructed plan of education, focusing on direct delivery patient care services. A clinical preceptor, acting as a mentor and validator, is available to masters students. This preceptor may be a nurse or physician. Both nurses and physicians need a clear understanding of each other's domain and have a willingness to mentor the graduate student and contribute to creative solutions of advanced practice. Often the advanced practice nurse is a 'loner' in systems, dependent on their own creative solutions to new problems. In this situation, it is even more imperative that collaborative relationships be established and used by the advanced practice nurse. The primary collaborative relationship must be with physicians as the overlap between disciplines becomes broader. This is not to say that the advanced practice nurse becomes a physician substitute or associate, even though some of the expanded skills once belonged solely in the domain of medicine. Collaborative relationships in planning and distributing care must be fostered with other therapeutic disciplines including physiotherapy, occupational therapy and so forth.

Scope of practice

Professional nursing has defined its standards of practice – standards that have undergone periodic reviews and updates in keeping with social change. Standards are the minimal expectations for all nurses in practice and act as a definition of nursing's practice (ANA, 1996; UKCC, 1992). Professional standards guide its members and determine the level of practice for direct care. Because practice is dynamic, so too must standards reflect contemporary practice patterns and future initiatives. The accountability for nursing's practice can be measured by applying standards. While standards are promulgated by the profession, they are interpreted by the public. In addition to using standards as a measurement of quality, they can be used in job descriptions, clinical ladders, performance evaluation, quality assurance systems, organisational structures and individual practices.

The scope of advanced practice nurses is evident in the degree of professional autonomy used by nurses. Autonomy in one practice may vary widely from other settings by nurses in advanced practice; however, the application of accepted standards will remain the same for both. The scope of practice is generally established by national or state authorities. Often the professional scope of practice as described by the professional organisation is consonant with the official authority, it may suggest higher levels for achievement. The individual advanced practice nurse is responsible for fitting practice into these national or state laws and is also accountable for incorporating ethical standards of care.

The characteristics of nursing's scope of practice include four defining principles – boundaries, intersections, core and dimensions (ANA, 1980). The boundaries, in response to social need, move outward. These boundaries may move at varying speeds, dependent on local need, interest and choice of the advanced practice nurse and are affected by scientific outcomes. Hopefully, the scope of practice is sufficiently general or broad so as not to hamper the movement of boundaries.

The intersections of the nurse's scope of practice acknowledges the overlap of knowledge, skill and activity of several disciplines. The overlap area is owned by those authorised to perform in it and the activity is within that profession's domain. For example, taking of a patients blood pressure is an overlapping function for several professions and the activity fits within their scope of practice. Intersections of practice often become the collaborative areas of practice, each professional with authority granted by their own domain. There is sometimes a temptation for one profession to supervise others when functioning in the intersections of care. Astute nurses will guard their practice domain through knowledge of their own definitions of practice – what is legal and what is not yet defined by authority, but has been accepted in the intersection of disciplines.

The core describes the essence of the profession. It is the basis for all of nursing's practice and includes the assessment, management and evaluation of nursing practice. Inherent in this process is the application of theory in understanding, guiding and solving dilemmas of care. Advanced practice nurses are leaders in application of nursing process – teaching, demonstrating and delegating to other nurses in the setting.

The dimensions of practice are within the scope of practice and represent the philosophy and ethical standards of care. The dimensions of practice include responsibilities, functions, and duties of care and also include the authority under which nurses are authorised to practice (ANA, 1980).

Thus, the scope of practice, authorised by the national or state society, is characterised by a core of knowledge and philosophy of care, and has flexible boundaries and expectations for collaboration with others.

Moving the Boundaries

Continuing evolution of the profession of nursing requires changing boundaries. As this evolution occurs, limitations can be removed or resolved through actual practice realities as well as through legislated policy decisions. Debates that review overlapping areas of interest between and among professions have focused on common work. The early work of Lewis and Resnick (1967), Spitzer *et al.* (1974), Sultz *et al.* (1980) and others was seminal in the beginning years of new roles. Commonalities of practice and overlapping areas of interest have recently been followed by confirming work of Safriet (1992), and Mundinger (2000). Several professions have common foundations, use education and research to further its practice and provide patient care equal to or better than others (OTA, 1986; Brown and Grimes for ANA, 1993). Territorial disputes have been prevalent for centuries and may not be resolved by using the same approaches in future.

When the nurse practitioner role emerged in the early 1970s in the United States, the clarification of professional boundaries took on a new dimension. Those who were pushing their boundaries outward were charged with practising medicine without a license or acting as a physician substitute. Internal and external members believed that the professional advance into others' territory was inappropriate for nursing. Indeed, throughout history, nursing has taken on more responsibility as its practitioners became more competent and population demands increased. How is taking on more responsibility different from expanding one's borders? The continuing evolution of the profession requires its members to expand programmes while generating new roles and duties. For example, nurses in critical care units have long taken responsibility for life-saving decisions and only recently have been granted authority for taking the action. Thus expanding responsibility and authority have become synonymous with developing advanced practice.

Since the early 1970s discussion has continued regarding the evolution of new roles. Today, however, there is ample evidence that advanced practice nursing delivers high-quality care, receives high scores in patient satisfaction, and is moving the profession into new levels of practice (OTA,

1986; Mundinger, 2000). It would be easy for nurses to mirror the work of the physician. If the only purpose in preparing the advanced nurse was to substitute for the physician, preparing nursing practitioners would be an easy task. We would recruit experienced nurses, teach them technological and procedural skills, and teach them algorithms of care for patient management. But this is not our mission. Simply put, 'we have a moral commitment to do more than imitate medicine' (Daly, 1997: p.6). Our vision is to advance the profession of nursing into new frontiers of practice, research and education.

The Reality

The continuing evolution of practice in cancer and palliative care nursing seems limitless. Distinction between practitioners, introduction of new technologies and application for future roles are all possible. Most nurses who practice in cancer care have a special sense of care needed and are experts at crafting that care according to patient need. It will be a challenge to distinguish between nurses working in cancer settings and nurses prepared in the cancer specialty.

While phenomena of concern for both may be common (e.g. a peaceful death), each may have a varying level of responsibility to deliver care, interpret findings and design new pathways. The earned clinical masters degree in the specialty of cancer or palliative care nursing should be the key element that distinguishes the practice and the individual. Through education, the nurse studies theories relevant to cancer and palliative care, and experiences faculty supervised clinical practice. Supervision is provided by faculty who themselves are cancer or palliative care specialists. This supervision includes constant, in-depth reviews of student competencies as they are applied in the field. These competencies include high level analytical skills in the application of cancer or palliative care nursing. The specific ingredients for the cancer or palliative care nurse specialist are thus:

- expert observational skills
- diagnosis of actual or potential health problems
- analysis of complex clinical and non-clinical problem
- selection and application of relevant theories
- determination of differentials in treatment
- development of short and long-range possible consequences

- communication of findings to other nurses, physicians, therapists, and all members of the care team
- interpretation of findings to patients and families.

Significant advances have been made by cancer and palliative care nurses in improving practice, assuming greater responsibility and authority for care and in legislating health policy which improves outcomes of care. Conceptualisation of the advanced practice specialty should focus on the body of knowledge that underlies practice rather than on the specific medical diagnosis or body part. For example, the breast care nurse would be a cancer specialist. While the specialty is cancer, the expansion of the practice of that nurse refers to acquisition of new knowledge and skills. Expansion of that cancer practice brings a wider base of knowledge and skills to the specialisation of cancer and it may overlap traditional boundaries of medical practice. The cancer specialist integrates research, practical knowledge and application in providing care to the cancer patient.

Programmes in graduate study, at masters or doctoral level, will need to develop curricula that prepare the cancer and palliative care specialists. This means a narrowed focus for acquisition of new knowledge and skill, using a broad repertoire from other disciplines and then applied to this specialty. Included in this advanced curricula must be a significant portion devoted to informatics. Knowledge from global resources becomes a strategic element in advancing cancer and palliative care nursing. Today, the internet links nurse to knowledge, nurse to patient, and patient to patient. All of this content contributes to the discovery of phenomena of concern for the cancer and palliative care nurse specialist (Ehrenberger and Brennan, 1998).

Rapid introduction of new chemotherapies for management and treatment of cancer have challenged the cancer specialist. Side-effect management has grown as a common responsibility of nurses. The future will undoubtedly involve greater knowledge and skill in chemotherapy management, along with a sound collaborative relationship with medicine. Nursing's ability to respond to patients needing palliative care fits squarely within nursing's domain. In fact, it is nursing that provides this care. The authority to do so, along with the responsible commitment, elevates the professional to new heights. Nursing leadership will come from cancer and palliative care nurse specialists, demonstrating high levels of care delivery and application of knowledge to that care. Goodman suggests that the freedom to take risks and carefully examine where boundaries should occur, fits within the advanced practitioner's role. She also stresses the value of research in nursing and its application both in improving practice as well as changing national policy (Goodman, 1998). All of this represents advancing nursing practice.

For nurses practicing in cancer settings, opportunities for advancing the work of nursing become a challenge and a mission. Despite the advances of nurses in cancer and palliative care, there is a continuing need to revise strategies and expand into new arenas. As nurse specialists continue to define the phenomena of concern for their specialty, all nurses working in the field will benefit. Thus, advancing practice in nursing will continue. While differences will always occur, the similarities promote a united effort worldwide. Emphasising the commonalties and glorying in the differences are the ingredients for nursing's future.

References

Albarran, J. and P. Fulbrook (1998) Advanced nursing practice: an historical perspective, in G. Rolfe and P. Fulbrook (eds), *Advancing Nursing Practice*. London: Routledge.

American Nurses Association (1980) *Nursing; A Social Policy Statement*. Washington, DC: American Nurses Association.

American Nurses Association (1992) *Defining Advanced Nursing Practice*. Washington, DC: American Nurses Association.

American Nurses Association (1995) *Nursing's Social Policy Statement*. Washington, DC: American Nurses Association.

American Nurses Association (1996) *Scope and Standards of Advanced Practice Registered Nursing*. Washington, DC: American Nurses Association.

Brown, S.A. and D.E. Grimes (1993) *A meta-analysis of process of care, clinical outcomes and cost-effectiveness of nurses in primary care roles; nurse practitioners and certified nurse midwives*. Prepared for the ANA Division of Health Policy. Washington, DC: American Nurses Association.

Castledine, G. (1982). *The Role and Function of clinical nurse specialist in England and Wales*. Unpublished MSc dissertation, University of Manchester.

Castledine, G. (1998) The Future of Specialist and Advanced Practice, in G. Castledine and P. McGee (eds), *Advanced and Specialist Nursing Practice*. London: Blackwell Science.

Daly, B.J. (ed.) (1997). *The Acute Care Nurse Practitioner*. Philadelphia, PA: Springer Publishing Co.

Davies, B. and A. Hughes (1995) Clarification of advanced nursing practice; characteristics and competencies. *Clinical Nurse Specialist*, 9(3), 156–66.

Department of Health and Human Services (1998) *National Sample Survey*. HSRA. Washington, DC: US Government.

Ehrenberger, H. and P. Brennan (1998). Nursing Informatics as a support function for oncology nursing research. *Oncology Nursing Forum Supplement*, 25(10), 21–5.

Elliot, P. (1998) Advanced Practice in the care of older people, in G. Castledine and P. McGee (eds), *Advanced and Specialist Nursing Practice*. London: Blackwell Science.

Goodman, I. (1998) Evaluation and evolution: the contribution of the advanced practitioner to cancer care, in G. Rolfe and P. Fulbrook (eds), *Advancing Nursing Practice*. London: Routledge.

Lewis, C. and B. Resnick (1967) Nurses, clinics and progressive ambulatory patient care. *New England Journal of Medicine*, 277, 1236–41.

McGee, P. (1998a) Specialist Practice in the UK, in G. Castledine and P. McGee *Advanced and Specialist Nursing Practice*. Oxford: Blackwell Science.

McGee, P. (1998b). Advanced Practice in the UK, in G. Castledine and P. McGee *Advanced and Specialist Nursing Practice*. Oxford: Blackwell Science.

Mundinger, M., *et al.* (2000) Primary Care Outcomes in Patients treated by nurse practitioners or physicians. *Journal of American Medical Association*, 283(1), 59–68.

Office of Technology Assessment (1986) *Nurse Practitioners, physician assistants, and certified midwives; a policy analysis. Health Technology Case Study No. 37*. Washington, DC: Office of Technology Assessment.

Royal College of Nursing (1988) *Statement of specialty*. London: RCN.

Safriet, B. (1992) Health Care Dollars and Regulatory Sense; the roles of advanced practice nursing. *Yale Journal of Regulation*, 9, 417–88.

Spitzer, W.A., D.L. Sacket, J.C. Sibley, R.S. Roberts, M. Gent, D.J. Kergin, B.C. Hackett and A. Olynich (1974). The Burlington Randomized Trial of the nurse practitioner. *New England Journal of Medicine*, 290, 251–6.

Steel, J.E. (1994) Advanced Nursing Practice. *AACN Clinical Issues in Critical Care Nursing*, 5(1), 71–6.

Sultz, H., M. Soelenzy, J. Matthews and L. Kinyon (1980). *Longitudinal study of nurse practitioners; phase I-III*. Hyattsville, MD: DPH Publication, No. HRA 80–2.

United Kingdom Central Council (1992) *The Scope of Professional Practice*. London: UKCC.

United Kingdom Central Council (1994a) *The Report of Post-Registration and Practice Project*. London: UKCC.

United Kingdom Central Council (1994b) *The Future of Professional Practice – The Council's standards for education and practice following registration*. London: UKCC.

United Kingdom Central Council (1995) *Implementation of the UKCC's Standards for Post-registration education and practice (PREP)*. Fact Sheet 6; Specialist Practice. London: UKCC.

United Kingdom Central Council (1997) *Position on Advanced Practice* (Press Statement 8/1997). London: UKCC.

United Kingdom Central Council (1999) *A Higher Level of Practice: Draft Descriptor and Standard*. London: UKCC.

United Kingdom Central Council (2002) *Report of the Higher Level Practice Pilot and Project*. London: UKCC.

11

Cancer and Palliative Care Nursing: the Influence of Policy

ANITA FATCHETT

Palliative care must be included as part of governmental health policy as recommended by the World Health Organization (WHO). Every individual has the right to pain relief, and palliative care must be provided according to the principle of equity, irrespective of race, gender, ethnicity, social status, national origin and the ability to pay for services (EAPC, 1995).

The Barcelona Declaration of 1995 underpins the philosophy which frames current palliative care nurse practice in the United Kingdom. First, it looks to ensure that the provision of such care is clearly part of all governments' health and social policy. Second, it stresses the importance of an equitable distribution of that care – a notion familiar to all nurses as expressed in the Nurse Professional Code of Conduct (UKCC, 1992). Such laudable aims cannot, and will not, however, be achieved by edict alone. In the real world of practical policy-making, the 'could' and 'should' will never become 'can' and 'will', until the proposed activity and focus are perceived as relevant, achievable and, most importantly, affordable, by those who make and implement policies for the nation's health.

Aims, however good and right, have to be translated from inspiring international declarations or professional codes – or even wishful thinking – to reality in practice for the many patients and families who face the profoundly complex and wide-ranging implications of life-threatening illess. The bridging of this gap between policy statement and effective implementation at street level NHS requires motivation, involvement, and continued enthusiasm from all interested parties – the public, the professionals and the policy-makers alike.

As such, Lugton and Kindlen (1999) aptly remind cancer and palliative care nurses of their professional responsibilities:

(1) To ensure that patients and their families receive the highest possible quality of care wherever and whenever it is needed.

(2) To work towards the development and maintenance of optimum levels of nursing care for the terminally ill.

These aims, like the Barcelona Declaration, imply the importance of nurse attention to both the context as well as to the content of care. As we are often reminded, 'Nursing does not take place in a political and economic vacuum. It is shaped and influenced by the prevailing political, cultural and socio-economic circumstances' (Fatchett, 1998b). Ackers and Abbott (1998) concur with this view, and acknowledge that while people become nurses because of a desire to care for others, 'their ability to do so is crucially determined by social policies. The ways in which services are actually organised and provided are determined not by the immediate providers of the services, but by government policies. Changes in policy-making impinge on the service providers as well as on the recipients of services'. Because of this, some counterbalance is surely needed to act on behalf of the wishes and needs of both patient and nurse.

During the period of the Conservative Governments' internal health-care market reforms, Finlay and Jones (1995) proposed 'in the business of healthcare provision, it is important that palliative care is identified, and integrated to the maximum for the benefit of patients, their care and the professionals'. This proposal remains just as relevant today under the current Labour Government, both for those with cancer or other terminal illness, as well as for palliative and cancer care nurses. As Fatchett (1998b) argued, 'it is increasingly evident that we will only gain the right to develop professionally under the current government, or indeed any government, if we take on the responsibility for influencing, creating and co-ordinating appropriate and modern professional nurse responses to the needs of the complex health agendas facing society in the 21st Century'.

Cancer and palliative care nurses, like the nursing profession in general, cannot afford then to be above or beyond the pursuit of two concurrent aims:

(1) The influencing, shaping and implementation of healthcare policy, with specific attention given to the equitable delivery of good quality cancer and palliative care.

(2) The continuing development of cancer and palliative nursing care practice at patient level.

These two aims are intertwined, and success in both areas is required, to ensure the continued maintenance and further advancement of these nursing specialisms within the policy agenda of the National Health Service (NHS). This discussion will turn to focus specifically on the many issues surrounding the involvement of nurses in the health policy-making process.

Nurses and Policy-Making: Some Introductory Thoughts

Over time the nursing profession has been accused of adopting a dismissive, even arrogant, 'hands-off' attitude to the business of policy-making (Ackers and Abbott, 1998; Clay, 1987; Haines, 1988; Salvage, 1985) It has often appeared to take the higher ground, focusing its energies instead on purer professional practice developments, while studiously avoiding the rough and tumble of political processes, which define both debates and decisions on scarce resources, and their allocation between one area of healthcare and another. Unfortunately, this perceived general lack of interest by nurses in the making and shaping of policy has often resulted in a side-lining of their knowledge, skills and ideas, in favour of those pursued by other (on the face of it) more interested and involved individuals. They, in turn, may have failed, or continue to fail (whether deliberately or not), to understand fully either the professional aspirations of cancer and palliative care nurses or the complex health needs of patients with life-threatening illnesses. As such, the arguments for directing ever greater resources towards cancer and palliative care may be made less strongly than if those directly involved were there to provide hard evidence of greater resource need from their experiences in practice. Indeed, it is proposed by the current UK government that 'the role and contribution of nursing to cancer care is vital at every level and at every stage of the cancer journey for those affected by cancer' (NHS Executive, 2000). It seems therefore appropriate to suggest that palliative and cancer care nurses should become active policy-makers. In this way, they can influence the direction of health policy for themselves and, hopefully, encourage the redistribution of an appropriate level of NHS funds in favour of the further development of their specialist nursing practice.

If nurses do choose to become engaged in the policy-making process, it is clearly important that they should familiarise themselves with its central concepts, allied activities and communication networks. This chapter now looks at the following:

(1) Policy as a concept.

(2) The policy-making process.

(3) The impact of policy on healthcare and nursing.

(4) 1979–April 1997: The development of the internal healthcare market reforms.

- The NHS reforms: Challenges to nurses and services.
- Cancer and palliative care services: How did these fare?

(5) May 1997 onwards: New government, new policies.

(6) *The New NHS: Modern, Dependable* (Cmnd. 3807, 1997).

(7) Cancer and palliative care nurses: The policy agenda.

(8) An agenda for action.

The aim now is to define both the concepts of policy and policy-making, and to determine their utility for those nurses who seek to advance the level of their professional practice, and to raise the standards of care offered to those with life-threatening illnesses.

Policy as a Concept

Like many of the words in the nursing lexicon, the concept of 'policy' is open to a variety of complex interpretations and nuances. Indeed, the potential for uncritical acceptance of the notion is considerable. Unless however, its attributes, characteristics and uses in practice are examined carefully, then any serious wish for effective involvement by cancer and palliative care nurses in the policy-making process is unlikely to be achieved. As Hill (1990) explains, 'Achieving policy change is never an easy process – to make a contribution towards this end requires not only knowledge of alternatives and commitment to putting them into practice, but also an understanding of what and how policy is made and implemented'.

As a concept then policy is widely used and applied in many areas of public life, for example industry, environment, housing, immigration, defence, childcare, the Prison Service, political parties, sport, religion, the voluntary sector, education and healthcare, to name just a few. As Colebatch (1998) described it, 'Policy is encountered in a wide range of contexts – different fields of action, different times and circumstances – and it would be impossible to cover them all'. Policy is created on both the international and the national stage, as well as on a smaller scale at local level, for example from WHO, to national, regional and local government, to the village cricket team and Brownie pack.

Levin (1997) set out a variety of usages of the concept, which he groups under four broad headings:

'Policy' as a Stated Intention

This relates to the taking of a particular action, or to the influencing or bringing about of a situation or change in activity. We can look at the stated policy intentions of the political parties in their General Election manifestos. For example, the Labour Party, in April 1997, stated its intention to remove the internal healthcare market structures and activities from the NHS were it to come to power on 2 May 1997 (*Health Service Journal*, 1997).

The Barcelona Declaration, as another example, looked to influence the shape of government policy by providing a framework of guiding principles which should underpin all governments' stated policy intentions for palliative and cancer care provision. Specifically for this discussion, we can refer to the Government's stated policy intention to combat cancer in the UK.

> We will develop and implement consistent national standards and develop the workforce strategy necessary to deliver high quality care. We will work with a range of organisations to look at how better to plan and share research; to provide the support and information necessary to enable individuals to participate fully in prevention and treatment decisions, and to set us on course to reduce the death rate from cancer and reduce by about 100,000 the premature deaths from this disease by 2010 (Cmnd. 4386, 1999).

Importantly for cancer and palliative care nurses, the Government has also stated its continuing support for the further growth and enrichment of the nursing contribution within the developing programme of NHS modernisation as set out in the 1997 White Paper (Cmnd. 3807).

> Nurses, midwives and health visitors are vital to delivering this bold programme of change. They are already playing key roles in establishing Primary Care Groups and Trusts, developing Health Improvement Programmes and service agreements and building integrated pathways for patients. As the new NHS develops we want nurses, midwives and health visitors to play a central part in implementing National Service Frameworks, and securing quality improvement through clinical governance.

Further to this, nurses are seen specifically as crucial to the delivery of a comprehensive service to those affected by cancer, and central to improvements in equity and access (NHS Executive, 2000).

'Policy' as a Current or Past Action

This concerns continuing policy activity, or some aspect of policy which has been developed in the past, and indeed, may still be effecting change currently. As an example, we could look back over the twentieth century and Labour Governments' attempts to reduce the inequalities in health within and between population groups. (Cmnd. 3852, 1998; Cmnd. 4386, 1999; Fatchett, 1994, 1998b). Similarly relevant are the observations and proposals for improvement and change in UK cancer care provisions and service as set out by the Calman-Hine expert advisory group in 1995. Further to this is the subsequent policy activity which has taken place, and which is continuing to happen, in establishing cancer centres and units across the UK in an attempt to provide a uniformly high quality of care both in hospital and community.

'Policy' as an Organisational Practice

This concerns the implementation of policy by the use of some established practices for an organisation, the rules and regulations, the ways things are done, and attitudes customarily taken by those carrying out the given policy imperatives. An example of this is the current Health Authority lead in the provision and shaping of care delivery and focus as set out in the 1997 White Paper (Cmnd. 3807, 1997). Another example is the heavy emphasis on the need for 'joined-up' thinking and activity across all areas of the Government's policy programme (Cmnd. 4836, 1999). This is evident in its attempts to fight cancer. The Government looks specifically for an integrated policy response from all potential contributors:

- A fundamental attack is needed on the risk factors which cause cancer, concentrating mainly on sustained reductions in smoking and improvements in diet, with action at all levels individual, local and Government is co-ordinated to secure maximum benefit.

- Efforts to combat the fragmentation and the variable quality of cancer treatment services, which have accounted for our past record of unequal survival patterns, must be stepped up.

Partnerships with cancer charities and other non-governmental organisations involved in cancer treatment and research are cornerstones of a high-quality approach to combating cancer.

Policy as an Indicator of the Formal or Claimed Status of a Past, Present, or Proposed Course of Action

In this case the term denotes a claim to status by virtue of being a product of deliberation and announcement – for example, by central government involving Cabinet deliberations and ministerial announcement. Such status has been given to the creation of Primary Care Trusts, the NHS Direct nurse-led reponse services, the Health Action Zones and Walk-In Clinics (Cmnd. 3807, 1997). The appointment of the so-called 'Cancer Tsar', Professor Mike Richards, by the Health Secretary Alan Milburn in 1999 (Watt, 1999), to oversee and to ensure the implementation of the Calman-Hine proposals, similarly implies the important status given by the Government in its policy efforts to combat the inequities in cancer and palliative care provisions still evident within the UK (Hogg, 1999).

As Levin (1997) explained, 'If a policy can successfully be labelled "government policy"... that policy will have a valid claim to priority over others not so labelled: in the allocation of money or other scarce resources. This can be seen in the process of deciding public expenditure'. Further, Levin explains that commitment and status necessarily often go together – 'decisions and announcements create commitment too'.

Ham and Hill (1993) similarly describe policy as a web of decisions and actions that allocate values, and, as a set of interrelated decisions concerning the selection of goals and the means of achieving them within a specified situation. The 1999 public health White Paper, for example, *Saving Lives: Our Healthier Nation* (Cmnd. 4386, 1999), is a good example of such a definition. It reflects contributions from a wide range of experts, and presents a structured policy for the nation's health. The White Paper states that, because the root causes of ill health are so varied, they cannot be resolved by focusing on health and healthcare alone. It acknowledges the need to tackle the potential determinants of ill health holistically. In the body of the White Paper, action is set out to be taken across all Government departments – and through partnerships between the various local and regional organisations in England – to reduce health inequalities.

Specifically, it describes cancer as one of the greatest health challenges facing this country, and draws attention to the variable quality of cancer services, and to the record of unequal survival patterns within the population. As the White Paper (Cmnd. 4386, 1999) puts it:

Among working age men unskilled workers are twice as likely to die from cancer as professionals. There is inequality between one part of the country and another. For example, women in the North West of England have a 33 per cent greater chance of suffering from cervical cancer than the national average. There is inequality between people of different ethnic origins, where for example, women born in the Caribbean are about 25 per cent less likely to die from breast cancer than other women living in this country. And there is inequality between the sexes, with women more likely to contract melanoma skin cancer, but men more likely to die from it.

In response to such appalling statistics, the Government looks to integrated action responses at all levels – individual, local and national, both in order to develop and implement consistent national standards and to secure maximum health benefit for all of the population. These issues have been clearly restated in *The NHS Cancer Plan* (DoH, 2000). The plan also sets out standards and targets to be achieved and suggests a mechanism (cancer networks) for implementation of the plan.

A word or two of caution on the policy thrust of these documents may however be appropriate at this stage. While health policy proposed by this or any other government may imply support, status and a strong claim upon healthcare resources, the reality is practice may turn out to be very different. The less specific a policy, the more options it leaves open when it comes to implementation. On the other hand, the more specific and detailed it is, the closer it is to being carried out and resourced appropriately in practice. We have yet to see if the required resources do follow the current Government's pronouncements on these wide-ranging and broadly inclusive health policies. Some may feel a little cynical.

The previous Conservative Government's *Health of the Nation* White Paper, for example (Cmnd. 1986, 1992), which was similarly broad in scope, was accused of having a general lack of specificity – not least in relation to a much needed financial back-up (Butler 1997; Fatchett 1994, 1998b). In addition, it is worth noting that the present Government's response to the issues around cancer, which have just been outlined, were subject to heavy criticism almost before the ink was dry on the White Paper. Senior cancer doctors were reported as warning the Government that its high-profile plans to tackle Britain's cancer survival record, claimed by them to be one of the worst in Europe, would make no difference to recovery rates (Coombes and Rowe, 1999). Reference was made, among other things, to the financial inability to prescribe the latest and most effective drugs, and to the under-funding of radiotherapy services. Criticism such as this creates doubts as to the seriousness of the Government's intentions to carry out its health policy programme and to fund it appropriately.

A policy then is calculated to achieve certain aims and goals in response to some problem or issue. Hopefully, it reflects both the contributions of those with specific expertise and knowledge of the issues, and the end product of an exercise in skilled problem solving. It involves the creation of an ordered response, drawing a range of varied activities and personnel into a common framework for action. Endorsement confers both status and authority upon it, and hopefully, but not always, the required resources (finance, people, time) to ensure its effective implementation. We will now consider the nature of the policy-making process itself.

The Policy-Making Process

So far then, the creation of policy seems to imply the deliberate and focused imposition of order for activity within and between organisations and personnel. It appears to emerge as a response to particular interests as expressed by any number of individuals whether at political, institutional professional or public levels. Policy is described as a product of rationale; a selective response to interests; the outcome of a process; and a reflection of power structures. As such, it is not surprising that the process of making-policy is often perceived as synonymous with politics and political activity. The words are often used interchangeably.

Politics is variously described as the study of institutions, rules, structures, norms, activities and procedures that are concerned with the allocation of resources. Colebatch (1998) refers to politics as being about the 'struggle' for a particular policy end. In turn then, political activity is about who gets what, when, where and how. For example, over the past century and markedly in this country, the political struggle has taken place (within the overall framework of a constitutional monarchy) between the competing political formulae of liberalism, conservatism and socialism – all of which have different perspectives on resource allocation for the benefit of the population. Despite all of the ideological differences, principles and nuances underpinning the focus of the policy direction taken, the national government of the day is seen as the final arbiter and decision-maker. It settles the complex political disputes and allocates resources within a framework for action. The policy-making process is the means used to achieve this end. In broad and simplistic terms, while politics and political activity are both labels to describe the steering of organisations in particular ways, policy and policy-making are described as providing order and organisational focus.

Wildavsky's (1979) definition of policy-making for example captures the slippery and complex nature of the concept. He states its aim to be to 'ameliorate problems through a process of creativity, imagination and craftsmanship'. Shaffer, too, describes public policy-making in almost lyrical terms:

> The public policy process is a multi-person drama going on in several arenas, some of them likely to be complex, large-scale organisational situations. Decisions are the outcome of the drama, not a voluntary, willed, individual, interstitial action. The drama is continuous (Shaffer, 1977).

Policy-making by government, for example in the field of health, involves a continuing and developing pattern of events; a 'drama' with participants from both within and without the sphere of central government playing their part. The process begins long before the announcement of any formal policy statement from government, and its implementation and development continues long after initial announcement and legislation. Some reflection back over the long period of the Conservative Governments' internal healthcare market reforms should help to clarify this particular point. Between 1979 and 1997, for example, the Conservative Governments' health policy objectives grew and developed with new and different goals becoming more or less clearly stated. There was also overlap and conflict between the many parties involved in the healthcare arena, for example general manager and doctor, Health Secretary, trade union and professional association, professional nurse and support worker, public and politicians, community health council and hospital trust, etc.

Ham and Hill (1993) have highlighted the overwhelming importance of negotiation and bargaining which have to occur throughout the policy-making process, the struggle and conflict between interests, the need to negotiate and to compromise which all add up to the reality of the process of making-policy. It is by these means that power and influence is gained and held, in order to pursue particular goals, and to shape health policy and the redistribution of resources in ways which reflect particular perspectives.

There are no fixed points for involvement but those who wish to take part need to seek out opportunities for themselves to influence developments and to push for emphasis to be placed on their particular issues of interest or activity. The development of the hospice and palliative care movement under the charismatic leadership of Cecily Saunders is a good example of such a move. Indeed, the subsequent attention given to this area of care demonstrates the continuing push by many players to place and to maintain cancer and palliative care at the centre of NHS policy-making. The Calman-Hine Report (1995), for example has, interestingly, spanned two different governments, clearly because of the persistent nature of these many different players at all levels who wish to influence and to maintain health policy in favour of the cancer and palliative care agendas.

In order to become involved then, Ham and Hill (1993) suggest a need to understand the following:

- The focus of different levels of any organisation – which is the appropriate level to approach?
- The decision-making structures – by whom and where are decisions made?
- The power relationships within and between groups – with whom to align – who to challenge?
- The connection between internal organisational power and structures and those of external contexts – which external players might be supportive or not?

Answers to these questions raised must be considered by all potential participants.

Colebatch's (1998) diagramatic presentation of potential policy-making players is also useful. He refers to six broad groups, all of whom may be involved in developing, implementing and evaluating policy activities:

(1) Those implementing policy – who are they?

(2) The 'authorised' decision-maker, for example the Government or Health Authority.

(3) Participants outside government, for example other statutory, voluntary or private-sector representatives.

(4) Other agencies, for example drugs industry, commercial sector.

(5) Other levels of government – select committees, House of Lords.

(6) International participants and influences, for example WHO, European Community.

Levin (1997) broadens this list in a more explicit and practical way, reminding us all of the various communication channels that could be exploited by nurses to secure support both internally to the NHS, and externally within the wider network of policy-makers interested in health-care delivery. These are:

- House of Commons, House of Lords;
- Cabinet and cabinet committees;

- Inter-departmental working parties;
- Government Ministers – briefing sessions from officials and advisors;
- Parliamentary questions by Members of Parliament (MPs) to Ministers;
- Select Committees;
- Consultation procedures – public enquiries, review bodies and tribunals;
- Media – television, radio, the Internet;
- Newspapers;
- Professional and other journals;
- Face to face meetings with local councillors and Members of Parliament;
- Pressure groups;
- Political parties and party conferences;
- Professional lobbyists;
- Machinery for monitoring, co-ordination and communication in the NHS;
- Letters to MPs, Ministers, Prime Minister;
- Letters to local authorities, regional and national bodies;
- Political, professional and business networks; and
- Social networks and contacts.

It is important to remember that policy-making is not just the remit or province of those who are most often formally identified as making and implementing policy, for example the politicians or perhaps NHS managers. As has been mentioned, there is an array of people with varying levels of interest in, and expertise on, different health policy issues, and with quite distinctive perspectives on offer. In addition, while the formal authority of government and its members in the two Houses of Parliament may be the authorised makers of health and social policy, in turn, the expertise of those with knowledge of and in practice is an equally important basis for participation in the policy-making process.

As Levin (1997) states:

It is not ministers and officials who look after sick people, educate children, run homes for the elderly, and dispense social security benefits. These tasks are organised and carried out by the other people in other organisations: in health authorities and trusts, hospitals, surgeries and clinics, local authority education, housing and social services departments, schools, colleges and universities....

When any health or social policy is adopted by government, its subsequent effectiveness and success will rely on the active support and involvement of those who are required to implement it from the centre, down to street-level practice and the general public. Indeed, without a continuing close relationship between all the interested participants, proposed policy activity may flounder or even fail, as for example with the introduction of the Poll Tax, and the workings of the Child Support Agency. Specifically then, nurses working in the field of cancer and palliative care need to maintain their vigilance and to be active in seeking the required resources to bring the Calman-Hine proposals to reality in practice. Without such efforts, other current and equally pressing healthcare agendas may take precedence.

As a conclusion to this section it is worth reiterating that entry into, and continued participation in, the policy-making process requires knowledge, motivation, continued enthusiasm, – and energy. It is unsurprising that many nurses feel they have too much to achieve in practice to become involved in the broader contextual issues of care. However, all professional nurses do have the potential and responsibility to provide those other nurse colleagues who are desirous or able to take up a more prominent role, with all the evidence and support they need to influence health policy in the desired directions.

'It is essential that cancer nurses who contribute at national level, are well informed and properly supported. They need to be able to draw on cancer nursing networks to ensure that important issues are raised and addressed' (NHS Executive, 2000). Without any doubt, palliative and cancer care, as in other areas of nursing, will have champions of change. But, as Saunders has argued on many occasions, everyone should do something to advance the care agenda, as every little helps (Saunders, 1999).

We will now turn to the impact of government policy on both healthcare and nursing. By doing this, we can begin to appreciate how very important it is to become involved in the making of health policy – much too important, in fact, to leave it to others.

The Impact of Policy on Healthcare and Nursing

The creation of the National Health Service ranks as one of the most successful innovations in social policy of this century. It represents a brave assertion of the equal value of human life, by ensuring that patients get the treatment they need, rather than the treatment they can afford (Cook in Fatchett, 1994).

Thanks to the NHS the population of the UK has been largely entitled to healthcare, free at the point of need for over fifty years. It is something of which we can be justifiably proud reflecting, as it does, a society expressing a practical concern for the health and well-being of all its members. The principles upon which it was established include

- the aim to cover the whole of the population;
- to provide equal access to people in need of healthcare;
- to be free at the point of use;
- to be comprehensive in cover;
- to provide services of a good standard for everyone;
- to be based on notions of public service;
- to be egalitarian in ethos; and
- to treat individual patients with respect as persons in the collective interest.

These principles, it is useful to remember, are very much reflected in the aspirations of the Barcelona Declaration (1995)

As a policy creation of the Labour Government, the NHS of 1948 was described as the most civilised thing in the world (Foot, 1973). A nurse writing in *Nursing Times* in 1948 expressed similar views:

> The great principle has been accepted. Never again need any of us suffer disease through lack of money. Let us be proud that a country still poor after a war has taken this courageous step. It will be responsible for its sick without question, because on the health of each member depends the health of the community. We are part of the service. This is a great time to be alive! (Whitting, 1948).

However, such enthusiastic support for the development of a national health service had not been universal (Foot, 1973). The Labour Government's health ministry, headed by Aneurin Bevan, had been involved in continuous arguments, struggles, conflicts of interest, negotiation and compromise – truly reflecting Shaffer's 'multi-purpose drama'. Conservative politicians on the Opposition benches, and many in the medical profession had been vehemently opposed to the creation of the NHS. It had clearly required all of the Health Minister's 'creativity, imagination and craftsmanship' (Wildavsky, 1979) to bring this major policy development to life.

However, despite all the initial wranglings, developments and changes to the NHS over the next three decades broadly reflected the support of the public, professionals and politicians alike. That said, by the late 1970s this consensus was effectively broken by the incoming Conservative Government of 1979. While providing reassurance as to the safety of the NHS in its hands, it embarked on the policy changes that would be necessary for the creation of a new business-like health service, one which it felt would be better equipped to deal with the health issues of the 1980s and the 1990s.

1979–April 1997: The Development of the Internal Healthcare Market Reforms

Under four consecutive Conservative administrations nurses and users felt the impact of major political and managerial policy shifts within the NHS, whether in hospital or primary care settings. Policy change involved the creation of an internal healthcare market, the separation of purchaser and provider roles, and the development of an underpinning ethos for care delivery which was both commercialised and competitive in nature.

The NHS Reforms: Challenges to Nurses and Services

The role of the professional nurse, associated values and achievements were seriously challenged during the period of internal market reform. While many did thrive both professionally and in practice (Fatchett, 1996, 1997, 1998b), others inevitably were unable to survive the demands made upon them. (Gillan, 1994; Salter and Snee, 1997; Thornton, 1995) The positive claims made for the reforms by government and other supporters which were designed to have benefited the user, the service and professional nurse alike, did not always meet expectations. The claims of the reformers to have listened and responded to patient preference were described as 'a well packaged ploy to cover up cost-containment, retrenchment in services, and a slow dismantling of the previously broadly based responsibility of the N.H.S.' (Fatchett, 1998b). Indeed, the promised notion of equitable care for all in need, implicit within the founding principles of 1948, appeared to have become badly dented (North & Bradshaw, 1997).

Cancer and Palliative Care Areas: How Did These Fare?

Neither field of care was immune to the inequitable effects of the workings of the internal healthcare market. Mason *et al.* (1996) in their research into the impact of the reforms made several interesting obser-vations. They found, for example, that hospitals and specialist palliative care units in the UK had survived the initial impact of the reforms with the majority coping reasonably well within the context of the quasi-market of healthcare. That said, their investigation revealed 'a varied and often contradictory picture'. The vast majority of hospices and special palliative care units had some form of contract in place to provide care, and the reforms were seen as having had a positive impact upon some specialist palliative care provision. However, researchers had also found considerable variation between hospices and specialist palliative care units in terms of their experiences of and response to the reforms, and surrounding the quality of relationships between purchasers and provider units. As such there were significant areas of concern that needed to be addressed 'before high-quality palliative care became available more equitably'. The observations and recommendations of the Calman-Hine expert advisory group highlights these points very clearly (Calman and Hine, 1995).

May 1997 Onwards: New Government, New Policies

The change of government from Conservative to Labour after 18 years offered the opportunity for a new administration with a different ideolog-ical vision both to halt and to redirect the processes of fundamental policy change and reform within the NHS. Prime Minister Blair, speaking on behalf of the newly elected Labour Government, referred supportively to the NHS in his opening address to the nation outside 10 Downing Street on Friday 2 May 1997:

> A new Labour Government . . . remembers that it was a previous Labour Govern-ment that formed and fashioned the Welfare State and the National Health Service. It was our proudest creation. It shall be our job and our duty to modernise it for a modern world.

This statement of intent for the shaping of a new and changed health service agenda pointed towards immediate policy activity. In the Queen's Speech at the State Opening of Parliament 12 days later, the government's intentions for change were stated:

> My government is committed to the development of the N.H.S., as a service pro-viding care on the basis of need to the whole population. They will bring forward

new arrangements for the decentralisation and co-operation within the service, and for ending the internal market.

The New NHS: Modern, Dependable (Cmnd. 3807, 1997)

The government announced its initial proposals for the NHS followed by a period of policy-making activity. Five months after the General Election the promised White Paper on the future of the NHS was published – the details of which have already developed and changed. It is against this which both public and professional will judge the sincerity of the Government's pre- and post-election promises for the health service as the millenium progresses. Central to all of the proposed changes envisaged in the White Paper was the removal of the lingering and negative effects of the internal healthcare market. These included:

● fragmentation of services;

● unfairness;

● distortions;

● inefficiencies;

● over-heavy bureaucracy;

● instability;

● secrecy; and

● a lack of true focus on the needs and preferences of the patients.

As the White Paper stated:

The internal market was a misconceived attempt to tackle the pressures facing the N.H.S. It had been an obstacle to the necessary modernisation of the health service. It created more problems than it solved (Cmnd. 3807, 1997).

By contrast, the new way for health policy would involve a rebuilding of public confidence in the NHS as a public service, one which was accountable, and based on the collaborative efforts of all involved (public, professionals and politicians), and open to the public and shaped by their views.

For nurses and nursing, the new health agenda appeared more sympathetic in scope, and gentler in ideology than hitherto. It potentially offered an opportunity to regain and to develop some new professional ground, not least for those nurses who have the professional skills and willingness to rise to the challenges being offered (Fatchett, 1998a, 1998b). The Government, however, was, and is not offering an easy ride for anyone. The striving for excellence, financial efficiency, effectiveness of care and care delivery, and clear proof of the value of all professional contributions to healthcare delivery were and are to continue. So what does it mean for cancer and palliative care nurses?

Cancer and Palliative Care Nurses: The Policy Agenda

Clearly there is a need for all nurses to play their part in the continuing developments in healthcare policy – not least to ensure that the voices of all those with life-threatening illnesses are heard and their needs met. This will involve a great deal of effort. Research carried out by MORI (1999) on behalf of the Cancer Relief Macmillan Fund, and based on interviews of sufferers, carers and patients' friends or work colleagues, has revealed massive gaps in care provision. As Nick Young, Chief Executive of the Macmillan Fund stated: 'For this particularly vulnerable group of patients and their carers ... it is now vital that we ensure their needs are more fully considered by those implementing the new N.H.S. reforms' (Hogg, 1999). The report highlighted the continuing need for a well co-ordinated network of practical, social and emotional support, as well as high quality healthcare, to help minimise the pressure on families. There continues to be a great deal of work needed to improve cancer and palliative care provision. Interestingly, Oxlade (1997) had warned nurses of the difficult and continuing challenge they faced in influencing both the implementation of the Calman-Hine proposals of 1995, and the subsequent directive EL(96)85 from the Department of Health.

As Doyle (1997) suggested, 'only when every hospital of say 100 beds has its own Hospital Palliative Care Team, and every district has its own specialist palliative medicine co-ordinator will we be approaching the ideal'. The MORI research above sadly reflects the need for continuing effort to achieve such an important goal.

So, how can palliative care nurses help to make this ideal a reality both for themselves and for their patients? How can they make their contribution to the health policy-making machine count? How can they bridge the gap between worthy policy statements of the ideal, and reality in practice for those with life-threatening illness?

An Agenda For Action

The important contribution of all nurses to the achievement of a modern and effective NHS has been made clear by the present Government (Blair, 1998). In addition, opportunities for professional advancement for those who have the skills and willingness to rise to the challenge are clearly available (ibid.). Cancer and palliative care nurses, like in any other discipline, need to ensure their continued participation in any and all such developments, both on behalf of their patients and for themselves. As it has been proposed:

> In the context of the national programme for cancer, everyone affected by cancer should receive care and support from nurses who are caring and competent, which is co-ordinated to provide a coherent service – from prevention, through primary care and screening services, diagnosis, treatment, rehabilitation and palliative care – and which includes close and seamless working with other professionals, the voluntary sector and social services and is aimed at securing the best possible outcomes (NHS Executive, 2000).

It has been proposed that action should be taken by the nursing profession on several fronts:

- the organisation, management and quality of care and services;
- workforce planning;
- education, training and continuing professional developments;
- recruitment, retention and career pathways; and
- leadership.

In order for palliative and cancer care nurses to address, and indeed to contribute meaningfully to such a broad programme, the acquisition or refinement of the following skills would seem both appropriate and very necessary:

- the ability to reflect on practice and to develop new ways of working in both cancer and palliative care fields;
- increased flexibility and creativity in care, appropriate to, and focused upon assessed local needs and circumstances;
- the carrying out and use of research;
- the ability to work collaboratively and in partnership with every-one involved in the broader cancer and palliative care environment; and

- an increased understanding of, and active involvement in the making of health policy.

By acquiring and developing these skills, palliative and cancer care nurses will not just be able to create ever more appropriate and effective care responses than now but will also be more able to influence a stronger policy interest in, and, greater financial support for, the care of those with cancer and other life-threatening illnesses. There is, however, another side to the equation. The nursing profession cannot influence and achieve such change alone. There is little doubt of the importance of all nurses' contributions both to the development of cancer and palliative care fields, and to promotion of these within the policy-making machine. At the same time, society and government also have a duty to provide nurses with the recognition they deserve – and patients with the care they need. The future development of high quality and equitably provided cancer and palliative care services in this country does not rest just within itself, but in a reciprocal partnership with the whole community.

References

Ackers, L. and P. Abbott, (1998) *Social Policy for Nurses and the Caring Professions*. Buckingham: Open University Press.
Blair, T. (1998) Blair to promise new era of supernurses. *The Guardian*, 8 September, 7.
Butler, P. (1997) Green Shoots. *Health Service Journal*, 23 October, 13.
Calman, K. and D. Hine (1995) *A Policy Framework for Commissioning Cancer Services*. London: Department of Health.
Clay, T. (1987) *Nurses, Power and Politics*. London: Heinemann.
Colebatch, H.K. (1998) *Policy*. Buckingham: Open University Press.
Cook, R., cited in Fatchett, A. (1994) *Politics, Policy and Nursing*. London: Bailliere Tindall.
Command 1986 (1992) *The Health of the Nation:A strategy for health in England*. London: HMSO.
Command 3807 (1997) *The New NHS. Modern, Dependable*. London: The Stationery Office.
Command 3852 (1998) *Our Healthier Nation. A contract for health*. London: The Stationery Office.
Command 4386 (1999) *Saving Lives: Our Healthier Nation*. London: The Stationery Office.
Coombes, R. and M. Rowe (1999) Blair's war on cancer is a sham, say top doctors. The *Independent on Sunday*, 14 November, 7.
Department of Health (2000) *The NHS Cancer Plan: A plan for investment, a plan for reform*. London: DoH.
Doyle, D. IN: Oxlade, L. (1997) Planning a future for palliative care. *Palliative Care Today*, 2(3).
EAPC (1995) The Barcelona Declaration on Palliative Care. *Progress in Palliative Care*, 4, 113.
Fatchett, A. (1994) *Politics, Policy and Nursing*. London: Bailliere Tindall.
Fatchett, A. (1996) A chance for community nurses to shape the health agenda. *Nursing Times*, 92(45), 40–42.
Fatchett, A. (1997) Delivering the Future: a new opportunity. *Community and District Nursing Association*, March, 13–14.
Fatchett, A. (1998a) Where Next? *The Yorkshire Practice Nurse Association Journal*, Winter, 3–4.
Fatchett, A. (1998b) *Nursing in the New NHS. Modern, Dependable?* London: Bailliere Tindall.
Finlay, I.G. and R.V.H. Jones (1995) Outreach palliative care services: definitions in palliative care. *British Medical Journal*, 311, 754.
Foot, M. (1973) *Aneurin Bevan Volume 2*. London: Davis Poynter.

Gillan, J. (1994) The Cull. *Nursing Times*, 90(3), 56.

Haines, S. (1988) Nurses for Sale. *Nursing Times*. 26 October. 84(43), 78.

Ham, C. and M. Hill (1993) *The Policy Process in the Modern Capitalist State*. 2nd edn. New York: Harvester Wheatsheaf.

Health Service Journal (1997) It's party time. 10 April, 12–13.

Hill, M. (1990) *Understanding Social Policy*. 3rd edn. Oxford: Blackwell

Hogg, D. (1999) Cancer families feel ignored. *The Guardian*, 7 July.

Levin, P. (1997) *Making Social Policy*. Buckingham: Open University Press.

Lugton, J. and M. Kindlen (eds) (1999) *Palliative Care: The Nursing Role*. Edinburgh: Churchill Livingstone.

Mason, H., D. Clark, N. Small and K. Mallett (1996) The impact of reforms on UK palliative care services. *European Journal of Palliative Care*, 68–71.

MORI (1999) Cancer families feel ignored. *The Guardian*, 7 July.

NHS Executive Department of Health (2000) *The Nursing Contribution to Cancer Care. Making a Difference. Challenging Cancer*. Leeds: NHSE.

North. N. and Y. Bradshaw (1997) *Perspectives in health care*. Basingstoke: Macmillan.

Oxlade, Lisa (1997) Planning a future for palliative care. *Palliative Care Today*, 2(3).

Salter, B. and N. Snee (1997) Power Dressing. *Health Service Journal*, 13 February.

Salvage, Jane (1985) *Politics of Nursing*. London: Heinemann.

Saunders, Cecily, Dame (1999) When you're 81, you don't care about diets. *The Times*, 8 June, 19.

Schaffer, B.B. (1977) On the politics of policy. *Australian Journal of Politics and History*, 23, 146–55.

Thornton, C. (1995) in P. Cain, V. Hyde and E. Hawkins *Community Nursing: Dimensions and Dilemmas*. London: Arnold, 110–43.

United Kingdom Central Council (1992) *Code of Professional Conduct for the Nurse, Midwife and Health Visitor*. 3rd edn. London: UKCC.

Watt, N. (1999) Cancer Tsar to end hospital 'lottery'. *The Guardian*, 28 October.

Whitting, M. (1948) *Nursing Times*, 3 July.

Wildavsky, A. (1979) *Speaking Truth to Power: The Art and Craft of Policy Analysis*. Boston: Little, Brown.

12

Developing Leadership for Advanced Practice Nursing

GILL COLLINSON

Leadership is a matter of how to be, not how to do. (Francis Hesselbein, 1999)

You may be forgiven for thinking that the concept of leadership is the latest trendy thing to hit the nursing professions and may ask yourself 'what has it got to do with me?' It is discussed in all quarters, across all specialties and regarded by many as being pivotal to the successful development of nursing in the twenty-first century. Indeed *Making a Difference*, the Strategy for Nursing, Midwifery and Health Visiting, published by the Department of Health in 1999, devotes a whole chapter to 'Strengthening Leadership' and states

> Aspiring leaders need to be identified, supported and developed. Senior colleagues have an obligation to spot and nurture talent, to encourage and develop leadership qualities and skills and to create a professional and organisational climate that enables the next generation of leaders to challenge orthodoxy, to take risks and to learn from experience. (DoH, 1999).

For the first time a substantial financial investment in clinical leadership programmes for nurses has been made, including programmes targeted at preparing nurses working in particular specialties, including cancer.

In this chapter I explore the concept of leadership and the relationship between leadership and the current healthcare context. I present different conceptions of leadership including those which I consider compliment the values and principles of cancer and palliative care nursing. I also argue that all specialist and advanced practitioners are those 'senior colleagues' referred to above and that they have an obligation to consider their leadership responsibilities and proactively seek to develop their leadership skills.

Context

Healthcare around the globe faces many challenges resulting from major social change. In particular:

- Demographic change
- Increase in available technology
- Rising public expectations.

Demographic Change

The aging population of the Western world provides a significant challenge for health and social care. The increase in the proportion of elderly citizens is creating a level of need for supportive care that we have not yet fully grasped. The risk of developing many forms of cancer increases with age and as palliative care services broaden to embrace patients with other chronic and debilitating diseases, the sheer volume of need will require nurses to reconsider the very best way of providing effective services of high quality.

Increase in Technology

Cancer and palliative care have always had a reputation of being in the forefront of utilising new healthcare technologies. Screening and treatment techniques along with specialist knowledge in utilising a range of technologies for symptom control have resulted in these specialties being recognised as innovative in both the science and art of healthcare. Even greater challenges occur when questions of whether the use of technology is appropriate require practitioners to develop within themselves clarity in relation to the values and beliefs that provide the foundations of their practice. At a strategic level nurses are becoming increasingly influential in determining what kind of services and treatments should be commissioned for a population based on assessment of local health need and evidence of clinical effectiveness.

Practitioners with such responsibilities may find themselves negotiating in highly political and emotive situations requiring not only clinical knowledge and understanding, but also knowledge and understanding of the policy and public health dimensions.

The rapidly developing field of gene therapy offers no end of future possibilities for cancer treatment, including those that are presently unimaginable. Yet their real presence as options for patients and their families is just around the corner and nurses need to develop a vision of what their contribution will be so that the preparations regarding practice, education and research and development needs can be made.

Rising Public Expectations

As our ability to detect disease and offer patients choices with regards to treatment and care increases the expectations of the population regarding what we can reasonably do has also increased. These expectations are not just regarding our ability to treat and cure disease, but how quickly we can provide a service that is tailored to individual need. Our patients are modern consumers, and when they can do everything from buy flowers to arranging a mortgage over the telephone or, internet, it is quite reasonable that they wonder why they have to visit the general practitioner's surgery to get a repeat prescription or wait days and weeks for test results.

It may be argued that public sector organisations such as the National Health Service (NHS) are slower to respond to social, cultural and economic changes than private enterprise. Whether this is true or not, the NHS modernisation programme is the British Government's strategy for re-inventing a huge organisation that finds itself ill-equipped to deal with the health-related consequences of twenty-first century social problems (Leadbetter, 1997).

Virtually every emerging policy impacts in some way upon primary, secondary and tertiary care, the commissioning and provision of services, and the monitoring of effectiveness and quality of care. *The NHS Cancer Plan* (DoH, 2000) provides the framework 'to deliver the fastest improving cancer services in Europe'. Its aims are ambitious and set new national standards and ways of working to achieve the goal. The nursing professions are recognised as key players in the modernisation of NHS cancer services and central to this new policy initiative. It presents a challenging leadership agenda for the profession and one cancer and palliative care practitioners must embrace if they are to successfully fulfil their potential. Not only will there be the inevitable opportunities to expand roles and responsibilities, but also the scope to influence what standards are set. For example, the way in which patients and carers are consulted and involved, services planned and the process of change implemented. Of critical importance to the success of the plan will be the need for nurse leaders to encourage and inspire colleagues to develop their knowledge and commitment to continuously improving standards of care at whatever point in the cancer journey they are involved.

Conceptions of Leadership

Since the early 1900s, the concept of leadership has been discussed, debated and written about widely. A plethora of theories have been developed, with many writers regarded as gurus, whose ideas and strategies can transform organisations. These theories reflect the time and social context in which they were written are therefore both susceptible to and responsible for changing trends.

Born to Lead

Early leadership theories focused upon discovering the personality traits of effective leaders, essentially developing the 'Great Man' or 'born to lead' notion of leadership. The trait theory proposed that someone born with particular characteristics would emerge as a leader for all situations. In particular these leaders were seen as being action orientated. Whether as politicians leading countries or generals leading men into battle, or pioneers exploring new lands, they led by doing and taking action. This conception of leadership identified 'charisma' as being an important trait for leaders, something you recognised when you saw it but found difficult to articulate or replicate. It generated the myth that great achievements are accomplished by the efforts of one extraordinary individual and that unless you were born with the traits to lead you could not learn leadership skills (Bennis, 1999).

Transactional and Transformational Leadership

James McGregor Burns (1978) uses the terms transactional and transformational to describe different ways of behaving, thinking or feeling in relation to leadership. The conception of transactional leadership can best be described as seeing leadership as a function. The transactional leader will see their relationship with followers as primarily being a process of exchange, whereby the leader provides either rewards or sanctions depending upon whether agreed expectations have been fulfilled to a satisfactory standard. The relationship is based upon formal, hierarchical roles and is concerned with the achievement of short-term tasks.

It also infers that the transactional leader has power by virtue of their position and can therefore 'command' followers to undertake tasks and 'control' the working environment, rewards and sanctions and is most often associated with leaders who are also managers. It is also probably fair to say that most public sector organisations, including the NHS, have developed like most large organisations, within a social and economic climate that valued security and stability, following two world wars. Authoritarian, militaristic and 'top-down' styles of management were the norm and were required to manage the enormous complexity of such national institutions.

However, by the 1980s, the global marketplace required organisations to respond to the rapid pace of change and emergence of new technology. Downsizing, diversity and flexibility became the new organisational watchwords along with the reality that there would also be less job security (Rifkin, 1996). Individuals would have to take responsibility for their own skills development and how they marketed and presented themselves. The old paternalistic relationship between employer and employee was gone, as was 'the job for life'. In this new environment employers have to attract employees with something different, if security cannot be guaranteed. In particular, employees are less likely to accept relationships based on authority derived from positional power and increasingly an organisational culture that is seen as empowering employees is regarded as being a crucial factor for organisational effectiveness.

The culture of an organisation evolves and develops from its purpose. The way it fulfils this purpose is through principles based on values and beliefs. Transformational leaders are primarily concerned with change and are able to communicate a clear vision of the future and the direction of travel by which to achieve the purpose or goal (Kotter, 1999). The transformational leader influences others to 'buy in' to their vision and follow them by virtue of there personal rather than positional power. They are persuasive, knowledgeable, well informed and credible. Kouzes and Posner (1996) further developed the concept of transformational leadership through research involving 5,000 participants, which they assert shows that 'leadership is an observable, learnable set of practices'. The current trend for transformational leadership stems from the need for organisations such as the NHS to undertake radical unprecedented change, which will only be successful if the workforce are committed to achieving it and involved in determining what the change will be.

While national policy has provided the broad framework for change, it will be for professions and organisations to interpret this for local implementation. The size and complexity of the NHS also means that it requires sound management to complement the visionary leadership. Burke and Myers (1982) and Kotter (1999) both argue that without vision organisations are doomed to repeat old patterns of working while without competent management the new vision may never become reality.

It also means that all levels of every organisation need competent leaders and managers. In essence it is every practitioner's responsibility to consider their role in the leadership challenge for their specialty or service.

Leadership and Nursing

A King's Fund Centre (1985) report suggested that there was a leadership 'crisis' in nursing in the United Kingdom. Since then there has been a visible investment in nursing leadership development by way of national, regional and local programmes. Yet the potential to liberate clinical practice and influence policy is still largely untapped, particularly among specialist and advanced practitioners who have not had either the opportunity or in some cases the inclination to broaden their vision beyond the day to day provision of a highly specialised service (Antrobus and Kitson, 1997).

Cancer and palliative care nursing has historically produced nurse leaders who have developed clinical practice, influenced health policy and raised the professional profile of nursing internationally. As a specialty it was one of the first to embrace the notion of clinical leadership through the development of clinical nurse specialists and expand the boundaries of nursing practice. However, I would argue that it is now this very specialisation that may potentially stifle the potential of cancer and palliative care nurses as clinical leaders and real agents for change in developing new and innovative services for cancer patients. Clinical knowledge and expertise are critical attributes for clinical leaders, however if cancer and palliative care nurses are to influence policy and practice, they are not enough.

By focusing on an increasingly specialised field of practice, that is site-specific roles, specialists run the risk of losing sight of the bigger picture. Such services have historically developed in a piecemeal way, often because of the passion and determination of an individual. However, if services are to be provided on the basis of need and located where patients can most readily access them, some services as we currently know them will need to change. Specialist nurses who keep abreast of the changing trends in policy and stay connected to what is happening within the broader organisation and local community, are more likely to be prepared for the inevitable change, rather than surprised by it.

Leadership Skills and Attributes

The literature about leadership and the many writers who extol particular skills and attributes provides anyone interested in leadership with life times worth of reading. However what must always be remembered is that leadership is essentially a function of perception. Whether you are considered to be an effective leader depends on how others perceive you. Their perceptions will be in the main influenced by their observations of your behaviour. So regardless of what your values and beliefs are, unless they are lived and evident from your behaviours, others will not necessarily perceive you to be the leader you think you are.

The Vision Thing

There are few authors that do not consider the need for leaders to have vision. Vision is one of the least tangible aspects of leadership and is often described in terms that make it mysterious and something unattainable for ordinary mortals (Kotter, 1999). It is, however, about setting a direction, of what practice, a service or organisation should become over the longer term. It is about having a broad goal, which is flexible enough to be adapted in the light of changing trends or new information. The vision does not have to be grand or highly original, but it must serve the interests of all the major stakeholders, patients, carers, colleagues and it must fit with the broader corporate objectives of the organisation.

Leaders gather lots of evidence, data and other forms of intelligence to find the linkages and relationships that will inform what the direction of travel should be; that is, it is about being strategic. Strategic thinking is consistently an area in which nurses seek development often considering it to be shrouded in mystery. It is however about facilitating meaning and crucially it also helps the leader explain their vision to others. For unless a leader can articulate a realistic way of achieving the goal and give cogent reasons as to why this should be the chosen direction, the leader will never see their vision become reality (Drucker, 1999). Sharing their vision also requires leaders to share their passion. Whatever their sphere of practice, whether it is clinical, research, education, management or development, the leader has a passion for achieving a better future and believes that they can make a difference. They challenge the status quo and search for opportunities to create, innovate and develop a better service, education programme, or body of evidence. They take risks and are willing to experiment and accept that they are likely to make mistakes and view disappointments as learning opportunities (Kouzes and Posner, 1996). If the managers' mantra is 'if it ain't broke don't fix it', the leaders' truth is 'when it ain't broke may be the only time you can fix it', because what was a successful formula in the past is unlikely to be so successful in the future (Zalesznik, 1998).

Integrity

Integrity is the foundation of lasting and effective leadership. Kouzes and Posner (1996) assert that:

> Honesty is absolutely essential to leadership. After all, if we are willing to follow someone whether it be into battle or into the boardroom, we first want to assure ourselves that the person is worthy of our trust.

Therefore the development of the relationship between the leader and the follower is one that needs to be nurtured and not taken for granted. The time taken in getting to know others and listening to their concerns all contributes to the development of a trusting relationship. The fact that people are constantly changing makes this a challenging aspect of leadership. But before this the leader must invest time in knowing and understanding themselves. Covey (1992) defines integrity as 'the value we place on ourselves'. If we are to articulate a vision and direction, we must first clarify our own purpose and values. By reflecting upon the choices that we make regarding our priorities and whether they are congruent with our values we develop self-awareness. By keeping the promises and commitments that we make to others, and ourselves we develop self-value. They are meaningless if we do not keep and value them and overtime others will cease to trust us and believe us.

Box 12.1 **Example**

A clinical nurse specialist was invited to become part of a group whose brief was to consider ideas and options for developing new ways of delivering a service in which she was a core team member. She believed that she had lots of good ideas to contribute, however every time a meeting was planned she sent her apologies because of the clinical workload. When she received the report of the group she considered many of the ideas to be impractical and found her own contribution to be limited. When she raised the issue with the manager and consultant involved she was shocked by their response – if you care so little about the future of the service that you cannot even be bothered to turn up to the meetings, what can you expect. They perceived her lack of attendance as lack of commitment. It is very easy to find oneself in this situation when you have what seem to be never ending demands placed upon you. Indeed the nurse specialist had probably not been proactive and taken the time initially to consider how important *she* thought it was to attend the meetings, in order to consciously make them a priority and organize theclinical workload appropriately. Instead she reacted entirely to the immediate clinical demands with the result that she lacked influence, became powerless and probably felt devalued.

Being a Role Model

If the effectiveness of a leader is determined by how followers perceive their behaviours, it is essential that leaders not only take the time to clarify their own values and articulate those values in terms of their vision, they must also set an example for others to follow. 'Walking the talk' is as critical for a leader's credibility as being regarded an expert in a particular field. If caring for and valuing individuals are values that you communicate to others, but you work long hours, never take holidays and do not look after yourself, you are not living by the standards you expect of others.

Leaders also recognise that complex change can create anxiety and inaction if people feel overwhelmed. In modelling the way they set achievable milestones so that an atmosphere of confidence is created and they always celebrate even the smallest achievement (Kouzes and Posner, 1996).

Motivating People

As change is the primary function of leadership it is essential that leaders are able to generate energy and motivation in order to sustain the change process through the obstacles and barriers which inevitably occur. As Kotter (1999) asserts:

> ... motivation and inspiration energize people, not by pushing them in the right direction as control mechanisms do, but by satisfying basic human needs for achievement, a sense of belonging, recognition, self-esteem, a feeling of control over one's life and the ability to live up to one's ideals. Such feelings touch us deeply and elicit a powerful response.

Empowering others and enabling them to act can radically and powerfully effect their whole lives. Leaders should not underestimate what a positive impact it can have, liberating people to be creative, take responsibility and develop in such a way as they aspire to new and even greater achievements. Effective leaders foster partnership working and build teams who are confident and willing to share with others (Kouzes and Posner, 1996).

Good leaders motivate by sharing their vision and passion and by regularly involving others in developing the vision further and working out ways of implementing it. Further they support employees' efforts to achieve common goals by providing feedback and coaching. Conversely where enthusiasm is stifled, ideas squashed or the credit taken by others, individuals can become, disillusioned, disheartened, demotivated and cynical. Change becomes a threat and their response to it is defensive. Such behaviours develop as a result of experience and being over managed and controlled, unfortunately an all to common experience for many nurses and others working in large bureaucratic organisations such as the NHS.

As change becomes the ever more constant characteristic of life in the NHS, leaders also have to motivate and encourage others to be leaders as well. Empowering others to develop their vision, energise others and implement change is essential within large organisations, because the complexity and pace of change requires multiple leadership roles, working together to achieve the bigger corporate goal (Kotter, 1999). Working in this collaborative way across departments and professions, not only has a positive effect on achieving the corporate agenda; it also makes for closer, more harmonious working relationships. More importantly still it is more likely to see patients receive co-ordinated care rather than situations where one department does not know what the other is doing.

Power and Influence

Many nurses consider the use of power as a negative and even distasteful. Yet power and influence are central to effective leadership. What distinguishes leaders is how they use their power. Covey (1992) presents three types of power, coercive power, utility power and legitimate power.

Coercive Power

The fact that many nurses see the use of power as a negative force is often because of their experience of being on the receiving end of someone exerting coercive power. Leaders who use coercive power creates fear in the follower, who believe that unless they comply with the leaders demands they will suffer in some way. Therefore followers put up with and acquiesce to the increasing demands of the leader. As the follower becomes increasingly unhappy their performance diminishes and thereby sets up a vicious circle. In many instances the cycle is only broken when the follower stands up to the leader or more commonly one or other leaves the situation.

Utility Power

Followers follow leaders with utility power because of the benefits of doing so. Covey (1992) calls it utility power because it is based on the exchange of goods or services, in much the same way as Burns (1978) describes the way in which transactional leaders approach their role. As described earlier this is the most common power relationship between employers and employees. Both coercive and utility power are most often derived from ones formal role within a hierarchy and are often referred to as positional power.

Legitimate Power

Legitimate power is of a completely different nature from those described above. It is the power that some people have because they are respected, trusted and others believe in what they are trying to achieve. Followers follow because they want to and most people can think of a leader who gave them an opportunity, provided a listening ear or in someway acted in a way that generated feelings of respect and a commitment in the other. Integrity and ethical behaviour are central to the values and beliefs of these leaders. Their power is never forced on others but rather it is invited as leader and follower pursue a common goal. Making a commitment to developing legitimate power is a long-term commitment for leaders who must invest time and energy in developing trusting relationships.

An individual's influence can be enhanced greatly by acquiring expert knowledge, information, access to resources, and promotions to positions of status. But unless the individual has invested in developing themselves and their relationships with others, achieving real sustainable change particularly in times of crisis is almost impossible without resorting to force.

Leaders require highly honed skills of persuasion if they are to have influence. Nurses with leadership aspirations often have little confidence in the persuasive abilities beyond the clinical arena. However, the skills and strategies used to influence patients and families are the same skills used to persuade those in more strategic decision-making roles.

Conger (1998) describes four essential steps for effective persuasion; establishing credibility, providing evidence, framing a common ground and connecting emotionally with the audience. The first two conditions are self explanatory, but the latter two are worthy of further discussion. In framing a common ground, those seeking to influence others must describe the benefits to the other. The persuader must take the time to discover what is high on the others agenda and whether their idea can help the other achieve their goals. It is about identifying shared benefits and creating a win-win situation and thereby making the idea so attractive to the other that they become as excited and as passionate about as you. If nurses are to see their vision become reality, they must be aware of and understand the broader corporate agenda and create a win-win situation for patients, practice and the organisation. In describing their ideas nurses must use a language that their audience can understand. The profession is already expert at interpreting the language of nursing and medicine in order to persuade patients, it must now become more competent at using the language of policy and management in order to influence the broader corporate agenda. In part, this can be achieved by nurses becoming more familiar with using the evidence generated from research, audit, clinical guidelines and management information. But to really influence nurses must convey their passion for their vision to the audience and connect with them emotionally as well as intellectually. We may think that all our decisions are rational and logical, but emotions are at play just below the surface of any situation. They convey the level of commitment an individual has to a particular course of action and the intuitive or gut feeling people trust in order to make so many decisions. Conger (1998) also claims that effective influencers are not only able to demonstrate their own emotional commitment but are able to accurately gauge the emotional state of the audience and sense when to adjust the level of emotion in the presentation.

In order to maximise their sphere of influence effective leaders must also invest time and energy in building wide networks. Networking may be considered to be yet another trendy buzzword adopted by nursing, but it is an essential part of any leaders toolkit. How one networks is closely linked to the other skills and attributes discussed. Integrity is essential and the most important thing about networking is to enter into it on the basis of what you can give rather than what you can get. Covey (1992) calls this an abundance mentality, which flows from a real sense of self worth and results in genuine sharing of recognition and reward. It means that you are confident enough to share ideas, contacts, knowledge, information and expertise without fear that you will lose status, position or power. It also means that you will receive something that is helpful to you in return, although it may arrive from an unexpected source. By going out of your way to find someone a piece of information, or send them a web address that they may find useful, you are developing your network in a genuine way. When you do need to ask for help people will be more than happy to, but remember to always end a request for help with an offer of help in the future. Examples of networking in cancer an palliative care service development are described in the next chapter in relation to delivering the objectives of *The NHS Cancer Plan* (DoH, 2000).

The Future?

There are many reasons and many theories why nurses have not fully realised their leadership potential, which are beyond the scope of this chapter. However, I believe that it is in part because some nurses are uncomfortable with the notion of power and do not value themselves enough to have the confidence to develop their personal power, but instead rely on the power of their job title or position. Once liberated from the restrictions of their position in a hierarchy, clinical experts can blossom into leaders who influence others beyond the artificial boundaries of organisational structure or professional pecking order.

In my own search for a model of leadership which aligned with my values and beliefs I stumbled upon the work of Robert Greenleaf and his theory of 'servant leadership'. What attracted me to this conception of leadership was that its primary premise was entirely congruent with the reason I originally became a nurse. Greenleaf (1970) asserts that servant leaders are servants first and then become leaders. As leaders their primary role is to serve their followers. For myself I became a nurse because I wanted to help others (be a servant) and was only interested in becoming a leader later in my career as I developed a passion for my practice and a desire to influence change.

Greenleaf developed the idea of the 'servant leader' having read Herman Hesse's novel, *Journey to the East*, an account of a mythical journey by a group of people on a spiritual quest. The central figure in the story is Leo, who accompanies the party as the servant and who sustains them with his caring spirit. All goes well with the journey until one day Leo disappears. The group quickly falls into disarray and the journey is abandoned; the group cannot manage without Leo. After many years of searching the narrator of the story comes upon Leo and is taken to the religious order that sponsored the original journey. There he discovers that Leo, whom he has known as a servant is in fact the head and guiding spirit of the order – a great and noble leader.

Greenleaf discusses the need for a new kind of leadership model, a model that puts serving others including employees, customers and the community as the number one priority. His work emphasises increased service to others, until recently a concept not regarded as trendy in our individualistic and materialistic society, a holistic approach to work, a sense of community and shared decision-making power. It seems to me that we are living in a time that more than ever needs servant leaders. As a profession we need to care for each other and those other col-leagues that we work with. The time for professional tribalism is past and if nursing is to continue as an attractive career choice we must treat nurses well, not just in terms of pay, but in how we value each others contribution. The organisations that we work for are, for many, the only community to which they belong, yet, they get bigger, more fragmented and impersonal. The 'Improving Working Lives Campaign', launched in September 1999, is a national policy initiative aimed at demonstrating care for staff working within the NHS. Building a sense of community within organisations and demonstrating care for the well-being of staff is critical to improving the reputation of the health service as an employer.

Finally our customers, whether they are patients, relatives or other users of our services, deserve to be treated well. Not just with the latest drug or surgery, but treated well as fellow human beings, at a time when they need our help and support. This is when we can be of greatest service. Those who want to serve first are different from those people who want to be a leader first. It is not to say that servant leaders do not have ambition or a desire to earn a good salary, with which to buy nice things, but this is not their primary motivation.

As nurses we have the privilege of holding in trust a unique body of knowledge and skills, the art and science of nursing, for future generations of those who will follow us as nurses and those who need our care. In his essay, *The Servant as Leader*, Greenleaf (1970) says that the best test for a leader is to ask themselves 'do those served grow as persons; do they while being served, become healthier, wiser, freer, more autonomous, more likely themselves to become servants?'

Being a leader can be a lonely business, it means that you are unlikely to be popular with everyone all the time. It is hard work and there are always obstacles to overcome in achieving the goal. But the buzz you get from the small wins you achieve with others, while working towards making the vision become a reality is so good it carries you through.

Leadership is always a work in progress – there is always another dream to dream.

References

Antrobus, S. and A. Kitson (1997) *Nursing Leadership in Context*, A discussion document. London: Royal College of Nursing Institute.

Bennis, W. (1999) The Secret of Great Groups in F. Hesselbein and P.M. Cohen (eds), *Leader to Leader, Enduring Insights on Leadership from the Drucker Foundation's Award-winning Journal*. San Francisco: Jossey-Bass, pp. 315–22.

Burke, W.W. and R.A. Myers (1982) *Assessment of Executive Competence*. Washington, DC: National Aeronautics and Space Administration.

Burns, J.M. (1978) *Leadership*. New York: Harper & Row.

Conger, J.A. (1998) The Necessary Art of Persuasion. *Harvard Business Review*, May – June, 85–95.

Covey, S. (1992) *Principle-Centered Leadership*. London: Simon & Schuster.

Department of Health (1999) *Making a Difference; Strengthening the nursing, midwifery and health visiting contribution to health and healthcare*. London: DoH.

Department of Health (2000) *The NHS Cancer Plan; a plan for investment, a plan for reform*. London: DoH.

Drucker, P.F. (1999) *Innovation and entrepreneurship*. Oxford: Butterworth-Heinemann.

Greenleaf, R. (1970) *The Servant as Leader*. Reprinted 1991. Indianapolis: Robert K. Greenleaf Center.

Hesselbein, F. (1999) *Leader to Leader, Enduring Insights on Leadership from the Drucker Foundation's Award-Winning Journal*. San Francisco: Jossey-Bass.

King's Fund Centre (1985) *Nursing Leadership: A Report of an International Seminar*. London: Kings Fund.

Kotter, J.P. (1999) *What Leaders Really Do*. Harvard Business Review on Leadership. Boston: Harvard Business School Press, pp. 32–60.

Kouzes, J. and B. Posner (1996) *The Leadership Challenge: How to Keep Getting Extraordinary Things Done in Organizations*. San Francisco: Jossey-Bass.

Leadbetter, C. (1997) *The rise of the social entrepreneur*. London: DEMOS.

Rifkin, J. (1996) *The End of Work; The Decline of the global Labor force and the dawn of the Post Market Era*. London: Putnam.

Zalesznik, A. (1998) *Managers and Leaders, Are They Different*? Harvard Business Review on Leadership. Boston: Harvard Business School Press.

13

Cancer Networks: Translating Policy Into Practice

CHRISSIE LANE, CLAIRE KELLY and DAVID CLARKE

Introduction

The chapters making up this book have focused on key contemporary issues which are worthy of the thoughtful consideration of all nurses who seek to advance nursing practice in cancer and palliative care services. This chapter will summarise the development of increasingly focused health policy in the cancer and palliative care field in England, and will then examine in some detail the impact of a specific piece of health policy, *The NHS Cancer Plan* on the future organisation and development of cancer and palliative care services. In particular the development of cancer networks and their contribution to delivering on the vision contained in *The NHS Cancer Plan* (DoH, 2000a) will be examined.

The developing relationship between health policy and research evidence was acknowledged in Chapter 11 by Anita Fatchett in her analysis of policy-making in the National Health Service (NHS). It is clear that that the rhetoric of evidence based health policy is becoming more of a reality in policy documents such as *The NHS Cancer Plan* (DoH, 2000a) and the *Manual of Cancer Services Assessment Standards* (DoH, 2000b). Fatchett exhorted nurses to understand and become involved in the policy making process, pointing out both the importance of influencing the health policy agenda, and the many opportunities which now exist to inform and influence that agenda. The strategy for development of cancer and palliative care networks discussed in the second half of this chapter addresses this issue in more detail. The challenges facing nurses who seek to advance practice in cancer and palliative care nursing are considerable but they are also an exciting opportunity for nursing to have a real and sustained influence on the development of services that will make a major difference in the lives of patients with cancer or chronic illness. Part of this influence will require nurses to work collaboratively with colleagues from other health professions. Shared skill development in the areas of assessment and communications skills may significantly enhance this collaboration. The developing 'cancer networks' can contribute to this agenda in a positive way.

Advanced practice nurses will also need to provide effective and innovative leadership if the potential of nursing, which was recognised by the Department of Health paper, *Making a Difference* (DoH, 1999), is to be realised. In Chapter 12, Gill Collinson examined the nature of leadership in nursing and pointed out the ways in which nursing leadership could develop to meet the challenges discussed above. It is clear that the type of leadership development which Collinson outlined, will be an important part of the nursing contribution to the modernisation and reform of cancer and palliative care services in both the United Kingdom and other parts of the developed world.

Before the specific development and role of cancer networks is considered it is important to trace the recognition of the need for reform of cancer and palliative care services in the United Kingdom from 1995 to the present day. While *The NHS Cancer Plan* (DoH, 2000a) recognises that cancer remains a major killer in the UK and sets out to provide a clear and comprehensive strategy to tackle the disease, it is important to note that the plan seeks to build on changes to service provision in cancer and palliative care which were set in train by the Calman-Hine Report (1995). The changes recommended in the Calman-Hine Report were given new momentum by further policy documents that are part of an overall strategy to modernise and reform the National Health Service in the United Kingdom. These policy documents, *The New NHS: Modern, Dependable* (DoH, 1997), *Making a Difference* (DoH, 1999) and *The NHS Plan* (DoH, 2000c) were to provide the context for nurses to play a lead role in major reform of the health service in general and in reform of cancer and palliative care services specifically.

The Calman-Hine Report (1995) recognised the heavy burden of disease which cancer placed on individuals, their families and the health service. The report pointed out the large financial cost of cancer to the NHS and was concerned to note apparent variations in the incidence of certain cancers, differences in the existence and accessibility of cancer services; and in the recorded outcomes of treatment. The recommendations of the report were comprehensive and wide ranging, relating to improving prevention of cancers, access to early diagnosis, appropriate specialist care and treatment, and palliative care. Recommendations were also made in respect of improving the education and training of health care professionals involved in providing cancer and palliative care services. Perhaps most importantly, the report laid the foundation for a strategic framework for the structure and organisation of cancer services throughout the United Kingdom. The report suggested that the new structure should be based on a network of expertise in cancer and palliative care linking primary and secondary care. These networks were not to be about buildings but about collaboration between specialist service providers guided by lead clinicians linked to cancer centres. The primary purpose of the changes recommended was to:

> create a network of care in England and Wales which will enable a patient, wherever he or she lives to be sure that the treatment and care received is of a uniformly high standard (Calman-Hine, 1995, p.1).

Three levels of care were proposed to deliver on the recommendations made. These were:

- *Primary care services* with clear patterns of identification of those at risk, rapid referral for specialist assessment and diagnosis and consistent follow up to ensure the best possible outcomes for patients;
- The development of designated *cancer units* in many district general hospitals, staffed by clinical teams with sufficient expertise and resources to manage the commoner cancers. The services provided in the cancer units would be organised and co-ordinated by an appointed 'lead clinician';
- The development of designated *cancer centres,* which would provide expertise in the management of all cancers, including common cancers occurring locally, and also taking referrals from cancer units to manage less common cancers. Cancer centres were to provide specialist diagnostic and therapeutic techniques including radiotherapy.

The three elements of the proposed cancer services were to link in a fashion described as a 'hub and spoke mechanism', with the cancer centre at the hub or centre of the wheel and the cancer units and primary care services being linked to the hub by the spokes of the wheel. Palliative care services were recognised as playing a key role in supporting the individuals and families affected by cancer at all stages of their illness, and not just near the time of death. The report called for the further support and development of palliative care services and their integration with the proposed cancer networks in all areas, arguing that palliative care services should be available in the home or community, in the hospital and in the hospice.

The Calman-Hine Report (1995) made 14 recommendations calling on a wide range of groups and organisations to take action to implement the recommendations. Coming as it did at a time when the NHS operated according to an established 'internal market', the recommendations called upon, purchasers, providers, health authorities, government health departments, professional bodies – including the Royal Colleges of Physicians and Radiographers – and individual general practitioners to take specific actions to bring about change. While the report called for its recommendations to be implemented 'swiftly', no clear timescales or deadlines were set. The report acknowledged that some areas such as training of new cancer specialists and provision of diagnostic equipment may take up to five years or more. The report also recognised that decisions on implementation of the recommendations would have to take account of local circumstances but could be taken forward by networks to be established by the NHS Executive and the Welsh Office Health Department. In some ways the report, although offering a sound vision and recommendations for improvement in cancer services, appeared to place the emphasis for making the recommendations a reality on existing cancer services, without acknowledging the wider health reforms and investment in education and training of specialist health professionals which would be required to realise the vision embodied in the report.

The change of government in the United Kingdom in 1997 brought about a shift in policy regarding the structure, organisation and management of the NHS. This shift was expressed most clearly in the White Paper, *The New NHS: Modern, Dependable* (DoH, 1997). The new government was quick to acknowledge that the NHS was in need of rebuilding if it was to be able to deliver high quality care free to all at the point of contact, promised when the NHS was created in 1948. Indeed the 1997 White Paper claimed the NHS was in danger of failing the people of the United Kingdom. The much criticised internal market with its divide between purchasers and providers was to be replaced by an 'integrated service' which would be the mainstay of a modernised NHS. An estimated £1 billion would be saved by this removal of red tape, and that money would be invested in an NHS where national standards of care would be guaranteed. Cancer services were explicitly mentioned in the White Paper with the claim that everyone with suspected cancer would be able to see a specialist within two weeks of their general practitioner deciding they needed to be seen urgently and making a referral. The target for achievement of this 'national standard' was April 1999 for everyone with suspected breast cancer and for all other cases of suspected cancer by 2000. Significant in the White Paper was the commitment to develop national standards and guidelines termed National Service Frameworks, which would be evidence based. There was also to be development of a National Institute for Clinical Excellence which would develop clinical guidelines from analysis of the latest scientific evidence. Both of these policy intentions are met in part by the development of *The NHS Cancer Plan* (DoH, 2000a) and the *Manual of*

Cancer Services Assessment Standards (DoH, 2000b). The White Paper provided the political and beginning economic support needed to deliver the vision expressed in the Calman-Hine Report (1995).

The document *Making a Difference* (DoH, 1999), which examined ways to strengthen the contribution of nursing, midwifery and health visiting in the NHS, focused attention on the lead roles that nurses could take in developing and providing new services. In particular the report appeared to recognise and support the contribution that nurse-led specialist services could make to a modern and flexible service which was focused on the needs of patients and not the needs of the service. The development of the nurse consultant role followed rapidly on from the *Making a Difference* report. There is increasing recognition that specialist and consultant nurses could transform some patient services. This might include taking responsibility for early assessment, diagnosis and referral in primary care, and supportive and therapeutic care in secondary and tertiary care settings (Corner, 1999). These developments are also significant in preparing the ground for nurses to make a major contribution to cancer and palliative care services.

The NHS Cancer Plan (DoH, 2000a) explicitly recognised that while there was much to be proud of in NHS cancer care, that the United Kingdom survival rates for many of the major cancers lagged behind those seen in the rest of Europe. The reality of the cancer services in the United Kingdom failed to match the commitment shown by the staff of the NHS. Major inequalities in the health of different social groups were acknowledged, as were the continuing variations in the quality of care and treatment across the country for patients with cancer. *The NHS Cancer Plan* therefore sets out a comprehensive national cancer programme for England. The plan has four aims:

- To save more lives, through and increased emphasis on health promotion, disease prevention and early diagnosis and treatment;

- To ensure that people with cancer get the right professional support and care as well as the best treatment,

- To tackle inequalities in health that mean unskilled workers are twice as likely to die from cancer as professionals

- To build for the future through investment in the cancer workforce, through strong research and through preparation for the genetics revolution so that the NHS never falls behind in cancer care again (DoH, 2000a, p.5).

The NHS Cancer Plan (DoH, 2000a) sets new and specific targets for health improvement and development of cancer services. These include targets for reduction of deaths from cancer by one fifth by 2010, reduction of smoking by between 4 per cent and 8 per cent for adults and children by 2010, and for an improvement in diet based on increasing fruit and vegetable consumption, particularly in children and poorer adult groups.

Ambitious targets were also set to bring in an extra 1,000 cancer specialists by 2006 and unspecified but increased numbers of nurses, radiographers and other staff who contribute to cancer care. Additional funds of up to £570 million a year by 2003–4 were also promised to support the implementation of the plan. This brief summary indicates the ambitious plans for improvement of cancer and palliative care services in England, but how will these plans be translated into reality, and what role will nurses play in the modernisation and transformation of cancer and palliative care services over the next five years? The next section of this chapter examines the way in which two regions in England have been working toward developing a cancer network and bringing about improvements in services. The examination of the nursing response and involvement in the initial implementation should demonstrate the importance of many of the issues raised in the preceding chapters in this book.

What are Networks?

A network is a web of free standing participants cohering through shared values and interests. A sense of co-operation among self-reliant, decision-making peers will vitalise a network. Personal networking is as old as the human story, from tribal villages to military organisations, human groups have used whatever means at their disposal to communicate over distance (Sessa *et al.*, 1999). However, it is only in the past few decades that people have consciously used networking as an organisational tool. The shift from working within hierarchies to making and working in networks is stated as one of the ten major mega-trends shaping the future (Naisbitt, 1986).

The emergence of networks and the change from traditional hierarchical healthcare organisations is described in this way by the NHS Confederation:

> Networks offer a new option which is particularly suited to situations where there are high levels of uncertainty, a need to co-ordinate multi-professional and multi-site teams and where simple solutions of outsourcing or vertical integration fail to address the problem of how to co-ordinate complex activities (NHS Confederation, 2001).

What is a Cancer Network

The Calman-Hine Report (1995) first introduced the idea of networks within cancer care as a model to enhance quality and equity of care. Networks were taken forward by some health authorities prior to *The NHS Cancer Plan* (DoH, 2000a) as a legitimate process by which to organise cancer services and enhance professional collaboration. Following its election in 1997, the new Labour Government recognised networks as a model of working which could break down organisational boundaries and bring about improved outcomes through collaborative ways of working. This was the catalyst required for cancer services to be delivered in a more patient/user-focused approach to care and involved heavily those clinicians who were at the forefront of delivering care. The appointment of a National Cancer Director gave a focus and provided the leadership required to standardise working together in and between organisations to improve cancer services.

The formal adoption of cancer networks was announced in *The NHS Cancer Plan* which stated:

> Cancer networks will be the organisational model for cancer services to implement the Cancer Plan. Cancer networks will bring together health service commissioners (health authorities, primary care groups and trusts) and providers (primary and community care and hospitals), the voluntary sector and local authorities. Each network will typically serve a population of around one to two million people. (DoH, 2000a: p.93)

In essence, a cancer network is a partnership between many organisations which as a whole consider all aspects of a cancer service; prevention, screening, investigation and diagnosis, treatment, palliative care and reha- bilitation. The underlying ethos being that networks will promote clinically led care throughout the patient pathway. The development of cancer networks demonstrates an emerging culture in the NHS; one of working across boundaries in partnership with a variety of healthcare organisations which may previously have been regarded as competitors. This challenge is all the more significant when one considers that cancer networks are supportive, facilitative, service improvement organisations not independent statutory bodies and therefore they are required to improve cancer services through influence and persuasion as opposed to formal organisational and hierarchical power and authority.

Effective communication and teamworking are essential to the suc- cess of cancer networks and will require nurses with effective leadership skills and a commitment to team development. Nurses have historically demonstrated their ability to work beyond boundaries and have embraced the opportunities which networks have to offer (Burton, 2000; Cook, 2000; ENB, 2001). Cancer networks require that all stakeholders recognise the value of collaborative working.

The Cancer Network – From Rhetoric to Reality

Cancer networks provide a major opportunity for nurses in all areas to influence cancer nursing practice and have their voice heard both locally and nationally. The development of cancer management teams in cancer units, cancer centres and cancer networks has provided a vehicle for influencing and improving local cancer services and provided a new leadership role for cancer nurses. The make-up of the cancer management team comprises three significant roles; lead nurse, lead clinician and lead manager. The lead cancer nurse has a responsibility to promote the development of patient-centred care through the role objectives described below.

Box 13.1 Role of the Lead Cancer Nurse

- In collaboration with the lead clinician and lead manager the cancer services lead nurse is responsible for the effective delivery of cancer nursing.
- Advances the development and practice of evidence-based cancer nursing
- Develops and implements communication arrangements with nursing and Allied Health Professional colleagues within the network
- Supports and advises on the implementation of the national cancer services standards
- Encourages nursing involvement in research
- Supports the development of cancer nursing workforce, education and training strategies

(*Manual of Cancer Services Assessment Standards*, Department of Health, 2000)

The structure of cancer networks enables the voice of cancer nurses to be heard and strengthens cancer nursing leadership. The Cancer Nursing Leadership Pathway (Figure 13.1) illustrates how nurses from a variety of organisations have a unique opportunity to influence cancer nursing services. The Cancer Nursing Leadership Pathway enables nurses to influence practice both locally and nationally through a process of two-way

Figure 13.1   Cancer Nursing Leadership Pathway

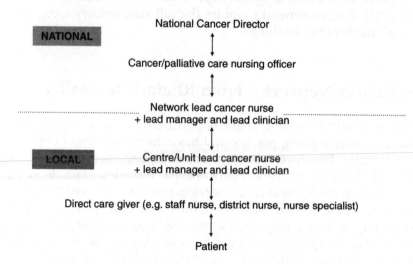

communication, allowing national policy to be influenced by local nurses and implemented with local translation.

Influences on the Cancer Network

There are now many national policy directives within cancer services that are influencing the direction and development of cancer networks, the following are key elements of *The NHS Cancer Plan* (DoH, 2000a):

- Cancer Services Collaborative
- Manual of Cancer Services Assessment Standards
- Improving Outcomes Guidance (through the National Institute of Clinical Excellence)
- NICE (National Institute of Clinical Excellence) Guidance on Cancer Drugs
- National Cancer Research Network.

All NHS organisations have a responsibility to work towards to achieving the objectives of associated with these key areas, and are encouraged to do so in new ways. The Cancer Services Collaborative (CSC), an NHS-funded cancer programme, aims to make improvements in the way cancer services are delivered and supports the wider modernisation agenda of the NHS. The principles of the CSC reflect the objectives of the cancer network, the principles of the CSC are:

(1) Certainty and choice for patients throughout their care journey

(2) Enabling everyone who provides cancer care to see themselves as part of the same system

(3) Reduce unnecessary waits and delays

(4) Provide a consistent, personalised service

(5) Making sure that patients receive the best care, in the best place from the best person or team. (NHS Modernisation Agency, 2001)

Nurses have been fundamental to the ongoing improvements brought about by the CSC supporting the development of patient-centred services. Nurse-led service improvements include nurse-led follow up clinics for breast cancer patients, development of systems to notify general practitioners of serious diagnoses and developing the role of nurse endoscopists. The CSC has demonstrated the unique contribution that nurses can make through using their knowledge and understanding of the patient pathway and the maze of services which confront patients through their cancer journey. The publication of *Manual of Cancer Services Assessment Standards* (DoH, 2000b) provides a framework for local cancer networks to assess the quality of existing and newly developed cancer services. These standards are based upon (disease) site-specific 'improving outcomes' guidance wherever possible and together with the specific cancer drug guidance being produced by the National Institute of Clinical Excellence, provide information and direction to plan, organise, deliver and monitor the effectiveness of cancer services across the United Kingdom.

National Cancer Research Network

Another important example of how networks are shaping the future of cancer services is the establishment of the National Cancer Research Network (NCRN). In April 2001, the Department of Health announced the formation of the NCRN, with the explicit aim to provide the NHS with an infrastructure to support randomised prospective trials of cancer treatment and other well-designed studies. The NCRN co-ordinating centre is based in Leeds and is being led by Professor Peter Selby. It is the intention of the network to:

- Improve patient care
- Improve the co-ordination of research
- Improve the speed of research
- Maintain and enhance the quality of research
- Improve the integration of research
- Widen participation in research.

By strengthening and accelerating the advancement of cancer research in the UK, the NCRN will:

- Take a strategic oversight of cancer research in the UK
- Identify gaps in current research and opportunities for future action
- Plan and co-ordinate approaches between funding bodies to fill gaps and take advantage of opportunities
- Monitor progress in implementing agreed plans and in achieving agreed objectives.

The NCRN will create a world-class health service infrastructure to support cancer research. It is a managed-research network that has been mapped onto the NHS Service Networks for Cancer Care in England. Thus strengthening the importance of networks as a model for improved cancer care (Selby *et al.*, 2001).

New Ways of Working in Cancer Networks

The NHS Cancer Plan (DoH, 2000a) has encouraged health professionals to embrace and value and importance of multidisciplinary working. The networks have supported hospital based multidisciplinary teams in meeting together; to remove boundaries and seeking to standardise the quality of cancer and palliative care across the geographical area. In essence, what this means for the patient is that regardless of where they live, they will be able to access high-quality care and will be cared for by an expert team working to uniform standards and pathways of care. The development of stand-ardised care across a network is facilitated at local level through network wide multi-professional groups known as tumour/site-specific groups and network nursing groups. The *Cancer Services Assessment Standards* (DoH, 2000b) document also called for the implementation of peer-review site visits as a key element of quality management for cancer services. These peer-review visits will be co-ordinated by (NHS) Regional Offices and will take place in every region throughout the country (DoH, 2001). Peer-review visits are designed to have a developmental and peer support function as well as the explicit quality management function, this approach further cements the collaborative and shared expertise approach to working in cancer services.

Human Resources and Workforce Planning

It is widely acknowledged that the cancer workforce shares the workforce problems of recruitment and retention with the wider NHS. The cancer networks are supporting the development of a skilled and competent nursing workforce in all areas of the cancer network. In the past there has been poor investment, lack of co-ordination and unstructured developments. Cancer networks in collaboration with the newly formed Workforce Development Confederations are to explore ways of establishing and maintaining a strong and skilled cancer nursing workforce. The Workforce Education Confederations for each region are also tasked with funding and developing education which is not only focused upon individual professional groups (e.g. nursing or medicine) but seeks to provide and foster multi-professional education which is grounded in the needs of specialist services in cancer and palliative care.

Network-Wide Education Strategies

The Manual of Cancer Services Assessment Standards (DoH, 2000b) emphasises the importance of education and training for all members of the multi-disciplinary team and the need for the planning and monitoring of cancer education. To ensure that all health professionals involved in cancer care receive appropriate training and continual professional development there is a need for a cancer education strategy at cancer unit/centre and network level. A network wide education strategy promotes consistency of education standards across the cancer network and takes into account the education needs of all members of the multidisciplinary team in a variety of healthcare settings, including nursing homes and primary care environments. Priorities for cancer education are highlighted through an educational needs assessment from which the education strategy is developed. This new approach to education ensures that the needs of staff who may have had restricted opportunities to access education and training in the past are addressed. The development of a cancer network education strategy has promoted the development and implementation of innovative methods of assessing and delivering cancer care education (Boal *et al.*, 2000). Innovative ways of educating and developing the workforce have been implemented through cancer networks and these are likely to influence the future of cancer nursing education.

Areas of focus for cancer nursing/health professional education include:

- Cancer competency frameworks
- Network-wide education strategies focusing on undergraduate and postgraduate education
- District nurse training in the principles and practice of palliative care
- Nursing homes education for palliative care
- Work-based learning initiatives as part of continuing professional development programmes or as part of higher education programmes.

Linking Primary and Secondary Care Services

The NHS Cancer Plan (DoH, 2000a) made explicit the importance of primary care involvement in cancer services. Cancer nursing traditionally focused on services within secondary care through the development of specialist roles in acute and generalist settings and the role of the community nursing staff in cancer care had been neglected. Health policy in cancer and palliative care has now recognised the value of all nurses in the community who have a significant role to play in improving cancer and palliative care services. Practice nurses, school nurses and health visitors are beginning to play a major role in the prevention of cancer through health promotion and health awareness activities. District nursing staff are increasing their contribution to the care of cancer patients throughout the disease trajectory from diagnosis to terminal care. The wider focus on the potential of cancer and palliative care nursing across primary and secondary care settings is firmly supported by *The NHS Cancer Plan* and, in addition the development of cancer networks has unleashed the potential contribution of many staff who may not have previously been considered themselves as cancer nurses.

User Involvement

The role of users in the modernisation of cancer services has been increasingly reflected in recent health policy. The Calman-Hine Report (1995) recommended that service providers take into account the views of patients, families and carers when developing cancer services. User involvement was specifically highlighted in *The NHS Plan* (DoH, 2000c), *The NHS Cancer Plan* (DoH, 2000a) and the Cancer Information Strategy (NHS Executive, 2000). User involvement in cancer services has been implemented to varying degrees, both informally and formally. While there is a lack of research in this area, one recent report has suggested that the development of user involvement has depended on health professional 'champions' that has resulted in a patchy, ad-hoc approach (Bradburn, 2001).

The participation of users in shaping health services is becoming mainstream policy. There is an increasing demand for NHS organisations and cancer networks (which also represent non-NHS organisations), to make user involvement a reality. There are a number of established users groups working at cancer network level that provide users with an opportunity to be involved collaboratively with health professionals in shaping local cancer services. From a user perspective, Bradburn describes the movement of user involvement in cancer services as a 'quiet revolution'. She eloquently states 'ordinary people at a time of extraordinary uncertainty and vulnerability have had Oliver Twist-like courage to ask for more – more communication, more accessible services, more pain control, more respect, more dignity and more emotional and spiritual support' (Bradburn, 2001). A key responsibility of the network lead cancer nurse is to 'ensure network wide user perspective informs the development of cancer services' (DoH, 2000a).

There are many methods that can be applied when involving users, for example patient satisfaction questionnaires, focus groups and advisory forums. Regardless of the method applied, achieving effective user involvement requires sustainability, inclusivity and a process that is valued by all stakeholders. Bradburn (2001) states that 'user involvement needs to be integral to the development and organisation of cancer services rather than running parallel to it'.

In response to the Report to the National Cancer Taskforce on User Involvement in Cancer Services (Bradburn, 2001) there has been a significant increase in user involvement activity at cancer network level. Cancer networks are being actively encouraged to engage with users, see them as equal partners in cancer services and seriously take into account their views. There is no place for tokenism in user involvement and this represents a huge culture shift from that prevailing in the professional led NHS. Cancer partnership/user groups have been developed in some areas and are recommended as an effective way of engaging users. It is recognised that this is new territory for many cancer leaders and users, support is therefore required to assist with the user involvement agenda. In many networks Cancerlink's Cancer-VOICES Project, which aims to give people with an experience of cancer a voice, is being enlisted to help networks to understand and meet the challenge of engaging users. Perhaps, most importantly, funding to support the personal development of users in cancer services has been earmarked by the Government. This is to ensure that the capacity is available to enable the development and sustainability of true partnership working. Service users no longer have to participate on a voluntary basis but are given financial recognition for their time and commitment.

Nurses are ideally placed to embrace this culture and power shift as they already spend much time with users listening and often documenting user's experiences in the form of audit and research projects as part of their day-to-day work. What must now be developed are skills and expertise to translate user's experiences into real service changes which are meaningful. This will present a challenge for all members of cancer networks but it is a challenge which will lead to improved and more patient focused cancer and palliative care services.

Challenges Facing Cancer Networks

A primary challenge for cancer networks is to influence hierarchical organisations and professions from a position of limited (organisational) power and authority. Managing change through influence at the network level requires strong nurse leaders who are able to work at a strategic level to positively influence the political agenda. Cancer nurse leaders require an ability to understand and manage the macro- and micro-politics and effectively translate policy to be meaningful to staff and patients.

Cancer networks are relatively new organisations that are reliant on the commitment and collaboration of other immature organisations, for example Primary Care Organisations, and Regional Workforce Development Confederations. 'Networks may stimulate creativity and innovation by providing increased opportunities for interaction of people from different disciplines and organisations' (NHS Confederation, 2001). The challenge for nurses in this environment is to articulate the voice and meaning of cancer nursing and ensure the patient remains at the top of the agenda as innovations in cancer practice develop.

Conclusion

Experienced health professionals know that policy statements such as those contained within *The NHS Cancer Plan*, do not always result in service improvements. However, the recent policy directives examined in this chapter go beyond simple calls for improvements and appear to focus on the infrastructure, working relationships and resources needed to bring about real improvements for patients. The skills, motivation and commitment of nurses to advance practice in cancer and palliative care were never in doubt, but in the past there has often been frustration at the apparent lack of opportunity to influence and lead specific service developments. Rigid hierarchical, professional and organisational boundaries, and politics contributed to the frustration. The Cancer Services Collaborative and cancer networks provide an important opportunity for health professionals to transform collaborative working from empty rhetoric to a concrete and workable reality. Nurses have been instrumental in shifting the agenda in cancer and palliative care from one that has focused mainly on the disease process to a vision of care which examines and takes account of the quality of care experience for people with cancer and their families. This vision emphasises psycho-social care, supportive care, effective communication and user participation. The newly developed roles of nurse consultant and nurse practitioner present unique opportunities for nurses to directly influence and improve the quality of care. These roles offer a model and opportunity to challenge the current modes of delivering cancer care, increasing nurses autonomy, and clinical decision-making skills. It is important to be clear however, that nurses at all levels can make a sustained contribution to improved services in cancer and palliative care, these nurses will look to advanced practice nurses to provide the leadership and direction to make the most of their nursing skills and knowledge. Nurses will be at the forefront of improving patient care, it is a role they are well equipped to play.

References

Boal, E., D. Hodgson, J. Banks-Howe and G. Husband (2000) A Cultural Change in Cancer Education and Training. *European Journal of Cancer Care*, 9, 30–5.

Bradburn, J. (2001) Report to the National Cancer Taskforce on User Involvement in Cancer Services, CTF (01), 11.

Burton, C. (2000) A description of the nursing role in stroke rehabilitation. *Journal of Advanced Nursing*, 32(1), 174–81.

Calman, K.D. and D. Hine (1995) A Policy Framework for Commissioning Cancer Services: A Report by the Expert Advisory Group on Cancer to the Chief Medical Officers of England and Wales. London: DoH.

Cook, L. (2000) Triple Integration Nursing. *Nursing Standard*, 14(52), 33–4.

Corner, J. (1999) Cancer Nursing: A leading force for healthcare. Editorial. *Journal of Advanced Nursing*, 29(20), 275–6.

Department of Health (1997) *The New NHS: Modern, Dependable*. London: DoH.

Department of Health (1999) *Making a Difference: Strengthening the nursing, midwifery and Health Visiting contribution to health and healthcare*. London: DoH.

Department of Health (2000a) *The NHS Cancer Plan: A plan for investment, a plan for reform*. London: DoH.

Department of Health (2000b) *Manual of Cancer Services Assessment Standards*. London: DoH.
Department of Health (2000c) *The NHS Plan: A plan for investment, a plan for reform*. London: DoH.
English National Board (2001) *Exploring the role and contribution of the Nurse in the Multi-Professional Rehabilitation Team*. Research Highlights No. 45. London: ENB.
Health Service Circular 21 (2001) London: DoH.
Naisbitt, J. (1986) The shift from hierarchy to networks in J. Lipnack and J. Stamps (1986) *The Networking Book*. London: Routledge & Kegan Paul.
NHS Confederation (2001) *Clinical Networks – a discussion paper*. London: NHS Confederation.
NHS Executive (2000) *Cancer Information Strategy*. Leeds: NHSE.
NHS Modernisation Agency (2001) *Cancer Services Collaborative Toolkit – Service Improvement Guide*. London: Hayward Medical Communications.
Selby, P., A. Palmer and R. Howard (2001) National Cancer Research Network. Briefing paper Leeds.
Sessa, V., M. Hansen, S. Prestridge and M. Kossler (2000) *Geographically Dispersed Teams* Greensboro, NC: Centre for Leadership Development.

Index